Living with Dying

Living with Dying

GRACE SHEPPARD

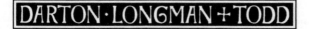

First published in 2010 by
Darton, Longman and Todd Ltd
1 Spencer Court
140–142 Wandsworth High Street
London SW18 4JJ

ISBN: 978-0-232-52783-4

A catalogue record for this book is available from the British Library.

Phototypeset by Kerrypress Ltd, Luton, Bedfordshire
Printed and bound in Great Britain by Thomson Litho, East Kilbride,
Scotland.

For Jenny, Donald, Stuart and Gilles
Who were there for me,
With my love

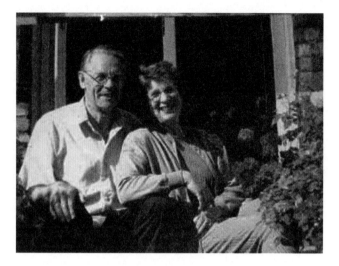

David and Grace Sheppard in their Liverpool days
(Photograph by Stephen Shakeshaft)

Contents

Acknowledgements

My thanks are heartfelt and go to:

My late husband David for his unconditional love, and care for me and for showing me how to suffer with acceptance and grace.

Jenny Sinclair, our daughter, who has been there for me and given me utmost encouragement, and for sub-editing my whole text; and to Donald, Stuart and Gilles – for their love, fun and practical help when it mattered most.

My brother John, and sisters, Hazel and Evelyn for faithful practical love, and many chuckles.

David's sister Mary Maxwell, for her encouragement and love; and for her example of courage with common sense, during her own double bereavement.

Liz and Frank Povall for their ever open door and deep and trusted friendship in all its forms given freely out of their own times of grief and loss; and for addressing all those envelopes.

Anita Cheung, Pat Crooks, Mary Cross, Brian and Pam Denton, Peter and Elizabeth Forster, Nick Frayling, Mary Gray, Ann King, Irene Perry, Jenny Plunkett, Joan Rayment, Alan Ripley, Ted and Audrey Roberts, Pat Starkey, Peter and Angela Toyne, and Desmond Tutu, all of whom have stayed regularly in touch and were especially close throughout this journey; and to all those many friends from the Mayflower and Southwark years.

To Stephen and Lorraine, Jed, Lucy and Isaac Broadbent and Mandy and Simon; for providing a gateway to heaven itself for me, in their home and workplace; a place of God's grace in which to rest and work without distraction, and with total understanding of what enables a person to flourish and be creative; and for all those cups of tea!

To Stephen Broadbent himself, for his imaginative and inspiring bronze memorial sculpture of David and Derek Worlock. Also for the bronze, *The Water of Life*, depicting Christ and the woman at the well of Samaria in Chester Cathedral cloisters, which has taught me so much about the friendship of Christ.

Brendan Walsh and DLT for commissioning this book.

Teresa de Bertodano for masterly editing and encouragement along the way. Helen Porter for her gentle, patient editing over the finer details.

Frances Sutliffe for her patient, sensitive and efficient transcribing.

Richard Buck for consistent prayerful, faithful and good-humoured spiritual direction in the early years; and for his friendship since.

John McManus for reading the whole text as it emerged, and for his constant encouragement; for his spiritual direction, and for his gentle, firm enabling of me in preparing to let David go. For sharing the struggle, and subsequently in bereavement years providing a rock-solid place which can only be described as the friendship of Christ on earth at its best.

To all who contributed so wholeheartedly to David's funeral and thanksgiving services.

All those involved in maintaining the physical and mental health of both of us, including Hanna McLuskey, Steve Briggs, Elaine Batts, Carol Makin, David Berstock, St John's Hospice on the Wirral, the Macmillan nurses team, and Marie Curie night nurses, and all in the NHS.

My neighbours in Melloncroft Drive for countless kindnesses, especially Noreen, Peter and Sue, Ian, Jim and Val, John and Margaret, together with Peter and Sylvia, Sheila and Ron who have since died and I trust are resting in peace now.

Friends at St Bridget's Church, West Kirby; especially Roger Clarke and Malcolm Cowan for their ministry.

Ruth Etchells for her constant encouragement to write this book, and for her ministry through her own book of personal prayers and meditations, *Just as I Am*, which has sustained me spiritually for more than fourteen years.

Mike Brearley for keeping in touch so gently and firmly.

John Ebdon and the Sussex County Cricket Club for their affection and generosity.

Godfrey Butland for his friendship and oversight of David's archive, and for his entry on David in the *Oxford Dictionary of National Biography*.

The *Liverpool Echo* for initiating the idea and seeing through the local appeal for a statue of David and Derek Worlock, and the people of Liverpool and others who donated money and time to see it unveiled in Hope Street on Pentecost Sunday in 2008.

To those who offered hospitality to me so soon after David's death.

Ian, for carrying all those letters and cards. Mark for helping me to keep the garden in trim. Diane for aromatherapy. Pat and Linda for helping me to keep my house clean.

To all who wrote, phoned, prayed and visited during our journey together, and since.

It is risky to name names like this, but I decided to take the plunge. It has been a most humbling exercise. So I am sure there have been some glaring omissions. Please forgive me if so. I decided to leave out titles here as it is the people inside their roles that I have been privileged to know.

Above all I thank God himself and the Spirit of Christ who has been my constant companion throughout this journey and whom I know will be there when it is my turn to let go in death. Until then I am filled with gratitude for life and for friendship.

Foreword by Archbishop Desmond Tutu

When I first met Bishop David Sheppard, I was immediately struck by his imposing physical presence. This was a big man. Very soon thereafter I discovered that his impressive physical stature was matched by its moral counterpart. He had given up the much coveted honour of captaining the MCC cricketers on their tour to South Africa because he abhorred that country's apartheid racist policies.

I discovered that this was a gentle giant, caring and compassionate as he ministered in South London as Bishop of Woolwich, especially with the most vulnerable and marginalised. He went on to cover himself in glory as Bishop of Liverpool in his splendid ecumenical partnership with Roman Catholic Archbishop Derek Worlock. He seemed so indestructible; he seemed to be going to be there always. Then as it were out of the blue came the shattering diagnosis of his bowel cancer. For most of us to be told we have cancer is like a death sentence because we may believe that all cancers are terminal, though of course this is not always the case.

The news shook Grace and David. It would have been odd if it hadn't. They would henceforth experience moments of darkness and questioning, perhaps asking the perennial questions, 'Why us, why now?' – all evidence of our common frailty and vulnerability. But mostly, they faced an inevitable reality – we are all mortal and the one certain fact for all of us is that we are going to die; that in a real sense, we are all suffering from a terminal disease – with a calm acceptance.

We are indebted to them both in that they decided to accept reality, not grimly, not with a defeated resignation. They were going to walk this intimate journey as persons of faith, knowing that ultimately nothing, absolutely nothing, not even death could separate them from God's love for them in Jesus Christ our Saviour. In this deeply moving account, we are privileged to accompany two loving spouses as they live with approaching death not grimly, not in any macabre way. No, they let us glimpse their intimate moments, loving, crying, laughing, David's bed placed so he could admire the beautiful garden they had planted together outside his room. They enjoyed music together, and were thrilled by the antics of their grandchildren.

Most of us do take so much for granted don't we? As if we will always be here to enjoy it all – a glorious sunset, the smile on our baby's face, the love of one's spouse, music, good food, etc. There is a poignancy in everything when you know for certain that it might be the last time you experience this or that or enjoying it with your life partner.

Living with dying can be shattering, gloomy and sad but it can also be a grace-filled time of moments of shared stillness and intimacy, of laughter and joy and tears, and moments too of facing up to the reality of life's transience. Grace has welcomed us into this intimate journey over four years as David grew weaker and eventually died, helping us thereby to live with dying creatively and positively. We are indebted to her for gracious generosity.

Introduction

In 1940 at the height of the Second World War my mother, younger brother John and I moved away from London and the bombs. I was five years old and John was three. We exchanged the ten-bedroomed vicarage with no heating for a small labourer's cottage in a village in the heart of Buckinghamshire. The address was 32 Milton Keynes. My father, an Anglican clergyman, stayed behind to care for his first parish in Battersea and to continue his duties as an Air Raid Warden. He subsequently became a padre, posted abroad with the British Army on the Rhine. He was awarded the MBE for his services.

During this time the family struggled. My mother was an asthma sufferer, and there was little money coming in. We were isolated from friends and family and, in those days, Milton Keynes was a small village. I attended the local school, which consisted of under twenty pupils aged from five to eighteen years old. My father was absent most of the time, returning occasionally like so many fathers in wartime. My mother would walk the five miles to the nearest shops at Newport Pagnell and back, pushing the pram which carried my brother, and the shopping. I walked alongside. It was during these walks I learnt to appreciate wild flowers in the hedgerows.

At seven years old in 1942, I was hospitalised for ten weeks with complications following tonsillitis. Pneumonia, jaundice and a collapsed lung took their toll. There was talk of putting me into an iron lung, which terrified me. With no private transport, my mother found ways of visiting me occasionally, but I treasured and still have the picture postcards she sent, which kept me regularly in touch with family news and with her love. After a spell in a convalescent home I was fit to return to normal life.

In 1944 we moved south to Haywards Heath in Sussex to a small house with a garden where we grew vegetables and kept chickens.

Flying bombs, or doodlebugs, were still appearing overhead. I have a vivid memory of holding my breath when at day school one day, and the gravelly threatening sound of the doodlebug's engine overhead stopped. I wondered if it would fall on me or on my mother ten minutes away, who was pregnant with my sister Hazel. My youngest sister Evelyn arrived in 1949.

In 1948 I went to Wadhurst College in Sussex, as a boarder. I was an average all-rounder, excelling in music and sport. In 1953 I gained entrance to Homerton College in Cambridge to train as a nursery school teacher and later became Senior Student. I qualified in 1955 and began to teach.

While in Cambridge I met and fell in love with David Sheppard and he with me. David was born in Reigate in Surrey and later became a pupil at Sherborne School in Dorset. His father, a solicitor who had served with the British Army in Salonika, had died from a kidney disease when David was eight years old and his sister Mary was fifteen. His widowed mother moved with the family to Slinfold in Sussex. He was a history graduate of Trinity Hall, and had returned to Cambridge to train for the Church of England ministry at Ridley Hall theological college. By this time he had done two years of National Service in the army with the Royal Sussex Regiment. He had also been selected to play cricket for England in the Test team.

We became engaged in March 1956 and married the following year on 19 June in All Saints Church in Lindfield, Sussex, during a thunderstorm, and in the middle of a heatwave. Our first home was in rooms in Islington where David was serving his first curacy under Maurice Wood, who later became Bishop of Norwich. That same year we moved to a flat in Canning Town in East London where David had been invited by the Bishop of Barking to resurrect the ailing Dockland Settlement No 1 as its warden. In 1962 our daughter Jenny was born, to our great joy. Three years later I was diagnosed with cancer of the ovaries and underwent radiotherapy. David became my faithful carer.

In 1969, David was invited by the Bishop Southwark, Mervyn Stockwood, to become the next Bishop of Woolwich, following John Robinson of *Honest to God* fame. He was consecrated by Archbishop Michael Ramsay in Southwark Cathedral and we moved to Peckham in South London. Six years later a letter from the Prime Minister invited David to become the next Bishop of Liverpool. He was installed in Liverpool Cathedral on 11 June 1975, St Barnabas' Day. We remained in Liverpool until David's retirement twenty-two years later in September 1997. During that period our daughter Jenny married Donald Sinclair from Glasgow and the Isle of Barra. They have two sons, Stuart and Gilles.

On retirement, we decided to remain in the north-west of England and settled on the Wirral. A year later, in 1998, we became grandparents. Then my father died. Nevertheless, we stayed in the north-west of England and had four idyllic years there until David's diagnosis of bowel cancer in the spring of 2001. It was my turn to care for him.

Much of this book deals with our experience of the subsequent four years. It is a personal account from the carer's point of view. My greatest dread was of losing David in death. This happened in 2005. Even now I stand back and marvel at the way I was upheld through his very public decline. Our forty-eight years of marriage contained a series of callings for each of us which tested our love and our faith commitment to the limit.

In looking at the way of David's passing in these pages I want to draw out some of the wonder of what has sustained me in these bereavement years. This has involved friendship at many levels. After David's death I decided to remain in the home and garden we created together, and in a community and neighbourhood that had given us so much friendship and support during his illness.

After his first operation, David encouraged me to keep a long-standing commitment to lead a conference for clergy spouses in Chester Diocese on the subject of 'The Friendship of Christ'. It was during this conference that it was suggested that the thoughts I had shared should be published.

I first became interested in pursuing this subject of friendship when working on my second book, *Pits and Pedestals*. David's close friend and Roman Catholic colleague in Liverpool, Archbishop Derek Worlock, had encouraged my writing and knew of my need for a quiet place to complete the book away from the bustle of Bishop's Lodge. He sent me a note, offering a desk in a room in Archbishop's House under ten minutes away. His note finished with the words, 'In the Friendship of Christ'. I was touched by his thoughtfulness and its practical outworking.

I began a third book on the subject with David's support. While putting aside two days to prepare a synopsis for Darton, Longman and Todd, something important happened to change my plan. On the first day, I received a phone call saying that a friend lay dying in a Liverpool hospital, and would I visit. The next day the front doorbell rang. It was a neighbour who had lost her husband and called for a chat. It was clear that I had to put my pen down and instead concentrate on doing friendship. The writing would have to wait. Then my mother's retirement home closed and, aged eighty-nine, she came to live at a nursing home near us on the Wirral. Shortly after this came the blow of David's diagnosis and priorities changed again.

There followed a challenging four years. My mother died aged ninety-two, while my husband showed us all how to live with cancer, with dignity, good humour and gentle acceptance, until his own death in the spring of 2005. We travelled a Via Dolorosa together which taught me much about God and myself. It taught us much about each other.

During that time I continued to write a daily journal that I had begun in 1985. Mostly I wrote last thing at night, but sometimes in the middle of the night and during the day. This journal became a vital part of my survival as a carer. It enabled me to note down an immediate account of what was happening, and to express what I was feeling during the ups and downs of the journey without burdening my beloved patient. My journal became a trusted friend and I have drawn upon it in preparing this book in which I have wanted to share something of what happened in the giving and receiving of love and friendship when life brought challenges which I thought were beyond me.

For both patient and carer there is a dynamic healing power in friendship. This has brought comfort, strength and that deep sense of belonging to me that I believe we were designed to experience from the beginning.

Like all creative arts, loving is costly. It involves sacrifice. It involves taking risks and having a spirit of adventure. That means effort, time and even pain in the releasing of those healing life-giving qualities that we seek. In the end there is joy. I experienced these qualities during the four years of David's illness. This experience continued in bereavement, and long after the death of

David, my parents and others. It has all been a surprising gift, and part of the boundless store of God's grace that he holds out to those of us who wish to respond.

I have looked again at Christ's last words to his disciples before his death and before their bereavement. His repeated plea was that they should love one another. Indeed it was a command, from a master to a servant. The meaning of love has been corrupted in recent times overemphasising the sexual aspect. Thinking about friendship has illuminated the love that I believe Christ was talking about.

During the twelfth century, the Benedictine monk Abbot Aelred of Rievaulx wrote on the subject of friendship. By all accounts he was a good friend to many of his fellow monks. He translated St John's words 'God is Love' to 'God is Friendship'. I found this to be an enlightening and even a thrilling concept – if perhaps a little controversial. Was Aelred constructing God in his own likeness, or was he inspired? Both perhaps? We shall never know.

On the last evening before his Passion and death, Christ had a lot to say to his disciples. Some of it was comforting. Some of it was revolutionary and radical. He said, 'I do not call you servants any longer. I call you friends ... Love one another ... that your joy may be full.'

Christ was calling for a profound change in their attitudes, relationships and approach to mission. There was to be a new way forward for them and a way of moving on after bereavement. It was to be a way of continuing to be creative and outgoing, but servanthood was giving way to friendship. No wonder the disciples were confused. They had travelled with a master who was leaving them. It was a further step towards change in themselves and in their relationship to Christ; a move towards maturity. What does that move towards maturity mean for us today?

Since beginning my search to find out, I have become increasingly aware of the wisdom of 'doing friendship'. More and more people in the developed world now prefer isolation and separation to mixing and sharing. We become too busy. The 'war on terror' has given us a different view on the way we regard each other. Fear stalks. Our defences are up. Cameras are around every corner. We find it more difficult to trust one another, in case we are speaking to an enemy instead of a potential friend. Our children can no longer play freely in the street or countryside without parents becoming anxious. Signs of affection towards them have become suspect outside – and sometimes inside – the family circle.

In developing the concept of God as friendship I can only scratch the surface of what this really means. Personal experience is vital and it is our own experience that informs us of the nature of God, alongside the facts of Christ's life presented in Scripture.

I hope to show from sharing a personal story that it is possible to see God a little more clearly by 'doing friendship', and by perceiving facets of the character of God in one another, in creation and even in solitude. I have found that the giving and receiving in faithful friendship has made all the difference to living with dying. We all have to die one day. The important thing is to be ready, and then we can get on with living. Knowing that we are all different, I pray that this story will enable at least one person to be less fearful of talking about dying and death with someone, to prepare, and then to enjoy each day as a gift. I long that this part of David's legacy may bring hope where there is despair, and joy out of sorrow, as it has for me.

The Parting

Our daughter Jenny sat on one side of the bed and I sat on the other. We held his hands. The curtains dividing the two rooms were drawn together. Our two small grandsons came and went quietly taking everything in. The nurse was like an angel of calm. She stood peacefully by ready to reassure and answer our questions. At one stage David stopped breathing and we asked her if he had gone. She thought that he had not, and he breathed again.

The words of my spiritual director came back to me with authority. 'Loving is letting go. The most loving thing you can do is to let David go.' Also the words of Christ to Mary Magdalene in the garden, after he had risen, came to mind. I thought I had let David go with my head and in my heart. But I had not told him. There was one more step to take. I had to tell him in case he could hear, so that he knew that I was not clinging on to him. Jenny moved over to be beside me. She said quietly, 'We'll look after each other Dad'. This would have warmed David's heart as it did mine. I leaned close and thanked him for so much in halting tones. Then, meaning it, I told him that I was ready to let him go – to the one who loved us more than we loved each other. In a few minutes he died. Jenny and I held each other.

****

It was just past 7 o'clock in the evening. The nurse standing by said that Jenny and I had said the two things that would have comforted and released him more than any other. His spiritual director had said in his final visit: 'He who can say, "In the end, God," has a strength that is impossible to fathom.' I believe that David returned home to God. He had been heading in that direction for some time, and now he was home at last.

At that moment I was given an awareness that his spirit had left his body, free from struggle and pain, and was, in my imagination, soaring high over the Dee Estuary. His body remained, lifeless now. The nurse laid it out with great reverence while we looked on, even talking to him as she went about her work. It was darker now. This was our Good Friday. We were left with David's body and with memories. His spirit was with us.

A while later at that same evening, aware that the family were still around and on the other side of the curtains, I thought again of our two little boys. I did not want them to be confronted with an empty bed without having the opportunity to see their Grandpa's body, now so peaceful, but devoid of life.

Before ringing the funeral directors to remove his body, I checked with Jenny and asked the boys if they wanted to come and see him. After a moment's hesitation, they came up with a will to his bedside. They were face to face with death for the first time and were not afraid. Sad, yes, but not afraid. David's legacy had already begun.

The boys have a firm foundation on which to build for the rest of their lives.

Chapter 1

From Private Commitment to Public Calling

In my end is my beginning.[1]

It was 19 June 1957 and there was a heatwave. Sussex had been playing the West Indies at Hove until the 18th, the Lords Test Match was due to begin on the 20th and I was marrying a cricketing clergyman.

The car drew up at the church. I gathered my long train and stepped out to take the arm of my father who was waiting in his top hat and tails. The dressmaker was there ensuring that her creation was as it should be, as she gently pulled a bit here and there. Straightening up and feeling excited, I looked for the doorway of the familiar and crowded church. For a moment I blinked. The door had disappeared. Instead all I could see, through the adrenalin, was a bank of 'holes'. Then I realised. The 'holes' were camera lenses. The press were in place and stood between me and my new life with the man I loved.

For a giddy moment I paused. Was this really what I wanted to do? Did I really want to move from a relatively private life to a public one? Did I want to be married to this man with all the extra dimensions of his being a celebrity clergyman? We had been engaged for fifteen months. There had been plenty of time to think privately about the various challenges ahead, to get to know each other better as human beings on a more intimate level, and to face lifelong commitment. We had become friends.

Even though I had had a taste of public life from being a child of the vicarage and from the moment the engagement was announced, I was aware, as I prepared to enter the church, of the pain of losing precious privacy. It was a little death. At the same time I remembered a phrase from the nineteenth-century Scottish theologian Thomas Chalmers: 'the expulsive power of a new affection'.

This doorway of camera lenses brought me up short for a moment. It was my last chance to withdraw. As well as being a doorway *from* something it was also a way *to* something. All I had to do was to step forward and go through that door.

It only lasted a moment, but that moment helped to galvanise my thoughts and to identify firmly what I wanted to do. There was no question. I loved this man. The flicker of fear disappeared and doubts withered. I stood for the cameras, picked up my train and walked through the photographers into the church to stand by David's side and take my vows.

I gladly and wholeheartedly let go of my private life, of my independence and of my name. We would become each other's next of kin, in place of our parents. I moved on from a kind of bereavement into a completely new life: and so did David.

Outside there was a cloudburst. We walked out of the church into a sea of umbrellas, smiling faces and heavy rain. Over the next forty-eight years we were to discover what this commitment entailed. I have never regretted my choice for one moment. It was, for both of us, a calling. It was full of little deaths and also full of life and new beginnings.

Honeymoon disaster

We spent our honeymoon in Italy. While driving to Florence several days after the wedding, I felt hot and not myself. The following morning I was covered from head to toe in spots. I had contracted a rare and virulent form of chicken pox, and was admitted to hospital. David was due to play in a cricket match at Leeds the day after arriving home. Caught between his two loves of cricket and his new bride, he offered to stay with me, and we discussed the options. So anxious not to cause a stir or to hold him back, I pressed him to return home so that he could play in the match. 'You go. I'll be fine!' I insisted. So he consented and went.

I was put in isolation in a semi-basement ward of an Italian hospital in Rapallo, knowing no one, without the language and with no prospect of visitors. Yet I was bursting with determination to get better and return to David and be the wife that I had dreamed of being.

There were bars at my window. I remember doing a pencil drawing of the view outside, which was a yard with a tree bathed in sunshine. But I left out the bars. This may have been wishful thinking. Nevertheless I was virtually imprisoned and not allowed anywhere until the spots and the fever had subsided.

The hospital nursing nuns visited my room less and less, leaving me with the medication to take when I wished. There had been talk of smallpox earlier which may have been the reason for this neglect. There were abortive visits to the hospital telephone at ground level to ring home. The line kept breaking down. I had to empty my own slops. Along the passage was another isolated woman, only she was demented and locked in. She shouted out *'Perche?'* ('Why?!') all day, beating on her door. It was a bit of a hell hole.

But there were moments of hope which came in surprising ways.

One day there was a knock on my door. It was an Anglican clergyman. He was clearly nervous of contamination as he closed the door with one finger and retreated to a chair in the far corner of the room and sat down. He had heard I was there, and came with an offer of help and the promise of prayers: a real angel in disguise. I shall always be grateful to him and also a little amused. His subsequent visits were made outside the window, pulling himself up by holding on to the bars, while passing books, and tickets for home, through to me. He was not a young man, and was anxious by nature. He was a lifeline.

Even the bars could not hold back the kindness. He represented that gift of connecting with the outside world, with other people, with a bit of God himself. The words, 'I was in prison and you visited me ...' came to life. I later devoured the stories of Brian Keenan, John McCarthy and Terry Waite, all of whom found ways of surviving enforced and unrelieved isolation and of maintaining their sanity in much more extreme and prolonged circumstances. The strength of the human spirit is powerful beyond our imagining. What weakens that spirit is to be cut off from each other. We read in their stories of the life-giving value of anyone or anything that enabled the hostages to feel connected to others. Even receiving a postcard from an unknown person made all the difference to Terry Waite and being given a radio by his captors became a lifeline.

These small gestures can keep the life flowing between people. Keeping in touch is vital for isolated human beings and for those who are pushed to the edges of good health and of society. If we fail them, two things may happen: either the human spirit will rise and fight to the death, perhaps at the cost of other lives too, or else it may die altogether from exhaustion. The light of life will be extinguished.

No wonder Christ spoke so much about being with us and not forsaking us. No wonder he urged us to love one another and to love our neighbour as we love ourselves. He wants us to survive. He wants us to thrive. He knows what happens if we refuse to do that kind of loving. He tasted hell for us and knows how to enable survival. Too many people are struggling in that place now. They need friends. They need a new kind of loving.

Leaving Italy behind I stepped off the train in Victoria Station only two weeks after the wedding, once again in my going-away outfit, and free at last from the dreaded spots and pumped full of adrenalin. David was there to meet me. So was the *Daily Express*. They took a picture of the two of us embracing through a window (I had to return to the railway carriage for the photograph). They also printed a picture of my nine-year-old sister who had been one of the bridesmaids, superimposed a spot on her cheek and printed the headline, 'The Spots That Spoiled The Honeymoon'. This was insensitive and hurtful for her. She had in fact recovered from chicken pox ten days before the wedding, and had no spots at all.

Never was there such a joyful reunion. David and I moved on, leaving that disastrous honeymoon behind. It was time to go forward.

As with most couples there were plenty of ups and downs, but underpinning them all was the knowledge that we were loved, not only by each other, but by God and by our families and friends. There is no better foundation. During our engagement we had learnt to be friends before being husband and wife. This had involved some discipline and resolve as well as an element of sacrifice and of letting go. It became an excellent basis for what was to follow.

Chapter 2

Early Days

*Go out and find friends among the young, among older people,
and those in society who are demonised and dehumanised … not
for the purpose of converting them to your beliefs, but for
friendship.*[2]

For a few months I began to build our new home at St Mary's,
Islington, where David was a curate. I threw myself into our new
life to make up for lost time. David was recalled to play for
England in the fourth Test Match against the West Indies in Leeds
and I went to watch the match. There was no time for respite or
convalescence. But I had not fully recovered. My self-confidence
had crashed.

Embarrassing physical symptoms of incontinence, shaking and
a feeling of unreality haunted me wherever I went. These were
unwelcome interruptions, and while I remained smiling and
cheerful on the outside, I felt guilty for upsetting things so early in
our marriage. I felt like a walking disappointment.

I kept all this to myself until the day I found myself unable to
breathe in a London Underground station while David was
preaching in St Paul's Cathedral. I shall never quite understand
what followed. I had only been home a few weeks. Leaning on a
fire extinguisher by the stairs in Holborn Underground station I
could go no further. I was gasping for breath and thought I was
dying. A kind man stopped and asked if he could help. I asked him
to walk with me to the street level. I thanked him and he went on
his way. In the congested street a taxi pulled up just outside the
station. Inside the cab were two parishioners from St Mary's
Church who recognised me. They saw that I was distressed and
invited me to join them in the taxi. More angels. We drove to the
medical centre at St Mary's where a doctor came to my rescue.

Was this coincidence? Or was this God coming to my rescue? To me it was a miracle and it is etched into my memory for ever. Here were three people who had had their eyes open and did not walk on by. Good Samaritans are still alive and doing their rescue work to the present day. In fact they are everywhere if we want to look.

My secret was now out; word went round the parish and I began to receive medical treatment. This was a difficult time for both of us in different ways. Grappling with disappointment, our love was not diminished. Rather it was tested. For David and his ministry, it was nearly time to move on anyway. Although he gave me no grounds to believe it, I nevertheless imagined that he must have been handling huge disappointment. My great fear was that he might want to walk away from our marriage and leave me. What I treasure is that he still treated me as a rational human being, able to discuss with him some of the big decisions that were needing to be made at that time.

Before our wedding, David had been invited by the Bishop of Barking[3] to become the new warden of the Dockland Settlement in East London which was in danger of closure. We had known that this move to Canning Town was on the horizon and that it would present us with a major challenge as a married couple. The centre included hostel accommodation for thirty residents, a church, a nursery school, a garden and other buildings. It was a place for local people and for all the family. It was to become known as The Mayflower Family Centre.

With a career as well as a marriage to consider, David had a tightrope to walk. My dignity was at rock bottom and so was my pride. We had been able to discuss the implications of the move. It was clear that, after a time of testing his vocation to this new job through meetings and visits and prayer, David felt called to this new work. It was also clear to me that, despite my vulnerability, I was called to be with him, whatever he chose to do.

We prepared to bid farewell to our friends at St Mary's, Islington, and venture into the East End, and a new community. I was both coming and going at the same time. We moved from curate's lodgings in Islington to the East End of London with the invaluable help of Hilary, David's secretary. I remember watching the piano being swung out of the window of our lodgings. I remember too the mixture of excitement and trepidation as we stepped onto the bare boards of our new home, which was a flat carved out of the hostel accommodation, on the first floor.

The complex was built on the model of a university college quadrangle surrounding a garden. We were the first married couple ever to have lived there. Previously there had been a single male warden, with students and others living in the hostel accommodation.

Our new home consisted of six rooms and a bathroom taken out of a hostel corridor. We put in a front door that locked, and fitted a knocker to preserve some privacy. We would often leave the door ajar to indicate that all were welcome. When it was closed that left its own message which was always respected. When living at close quarters with others, it sometimes becomes necessary to have ways of preserving some space and privacy that are easily understood and accepted.

We moved in August 1958, thirteen years after the end of the Second World War. Bombsites surrounded our building. They became playgrounds for the children who played football there, and who gathered round bonfires to be together and keep warm in the winter. Women met over heaps of clothes to sell and exchange, and to talk to each other. Bombed sites were their open-air community centres.

Gradually the builders moved in, new flats rose outside our walls. The debris disappeared. Our Centre now provided a meeting place throughout the week for young and old alike.

I was still unable to go out alone. Agoraphobia had taken hold; the fear of open spaces and public places. The Mayflower community were accepting and helpful, offering to keep me company, and help with the shopping as I was afraid of being alone outside the walls of the Centre. In the early days I would venture out across the courtyard and visit the clubs or sit at the back in church.

Here Peter, a young resident on duty, would greet me with a genuine smile and understanding beyond his years. He never tried to push me or persuade me to go forward to a seat nearer the front. Here was another angel in disguise. Peter connected with the stronger part of me and kept it alive. He trusted me to make my own decisions. This gave me space to help myself. He would joke, too, which I loved. Years later Peter was ordained priest, and is now a retired archdeacon.

This sort of kindness to me released David to carry on with his work when it could have been even more challenging than it already was. He was living with a wife who was virtually disabled, but he never once made me feel I was a nuisance. He believed in me and in my will to get better. 'You can do it' are wonderful words to someone who has lost self-confidence, and from someone who knows you well. David was young and innocent and often did not know what to do to help. It must have been frightening and disappointing for him and not a little frustrating. Nevertheless he was there for me. His patience and trust and his ability to get on with his work comforted me. He entered into my suffering with true compassion, and became a major part of my healing. Little did we realise the full implications of our vows on our wedding day to be there for each other 'in sickness and in health till death us do part'. I continued to grow in confidence, nourished by the loving acceptance of the community.

In 1962 I gave birth to our daughter Jenny with great joy. Pregnancy had agreed with me. This was a moment of transition. We became parents as well as husband and wife. Jenny was a very contented baby and she was to grow up with Beatles music playing loudly in the room above her bedroom where a young people's group met regularly. By this time I was much better, and able to function normally at home. Outside, it was another story. I needed someone with me when I went out. We were greatly blessed with several people who gave up their time to help me voluntarily.

At the end of 1962 David was given sabbatical leave and recalled to play cricket for England in the Test against Australia. This meant travelling to the other side of the world. Jenny was a few months old and David wanted us to go too as, in those days, families were encouraged to be there. Penny Cowdrey and Su Dexter were the only other wives who came. This venture was a huge challenge as I still could not cross a road alone. The team would travel earlier and separately so it would mean going by sea with Jenny, who was a few months old, and without David for four weeks. I decided to give it a go. Hilary, who was also Jenny's godmother, came with us, which made all the difference. We set up a temporary home in Sydney while David stayed with the team. We lived there for ten weeks.

Jenny celebrated her first birthday in Australia in extreme heat. At Christmas I had my first oyster, lunching with the Test team who had ordered a dozen each. Ted Dexter teased me, very gently, into joining the rest of them in ordering a dozen oysters for myself. I was hooked. The Australian adventure had all been well worth the effort though I had my moments.

We returned to East London for a few more years. When Jenny was three I was admitted to hospital for acute appendicitis which turned out to be ovarian cancer. The ovaries were removed, and radiotherapy followed. Once again David was my rock. We had the support of our families and the Mayflower community. A dear friend gave us some money to get away to a hotel for a fortnight following my radiotherapy treatment which had laid me low. This practical love and kindness enabled us to be together in private, to talk and to relax while gathering strength, and to be catered for for a change. Jenny stayed with David's mother; this two-week respite was as necessary for him as for me.

Sadly, the other four women in my hospital ward all died of cancer. Over forty years later I am the only one still here to tell the tale. There is no end to my gratitude for the gift of life. I feel a debt of gratitude to all those who stood by me in those years. It has made me very much aware of all those who struggle in their silent prisons and have no one to understand or care.

David and I stayed in Canning Town for twelve fulfilling years. From a challenging beginning we went on to discover that we were among friends. Fifty years later many of those friends still remain in touch.

We discovered that angels lived in dockland and were welcomed into that community with a warmth and hospitality that knew no bounds. They made us incomers feel at home, but not before we had put down some of our superior attitudes of coming to 'do good' and to 'lead'. We had corners that needed to be knocked off and a lot to learn and receive as well as a lot to give.

In his inaugural sermon in 2005, the Archbishop of York, John Sentamu, uttered words which ring loud bells for me after living in East London and in a different culture. He said, 'Go out and find friends among the young, among older people, and those in society who are demonised and dehumanised … go and find friends who are Buddhists, Hindus, Jews, Muslims, Sikhs, agnostics, atheists – not for the purpose of converting them to your beliefs, but for friendship.'

'Go and *find* friends', not 'Go and *make* friends'. The friends are already there. They are waiting, getting on with their lives, and reaching out with a welcome. Not to convert, 'but for friendship'. This may be controversial among certain groups of Christians who are too keen to proselytise, which can give rise to the suspicion of ulterior motives in their offers of friendship. True unconditional friendship is part of God's grace. It is catching. This does not prevent Christ from being named. Taken at face value, true friendship can lead into the reality of God anyway. We will meet God face to face in the encounter. But we have to reach out too. How else can we shake hands in genuine friendship?

David and I had arrived as strangers entering an alien culture, yet we shared a common humanity at a deep level. Those years in East London were part of our training ground for the future. Coming from private school backgrounds, we needed educating further. We were welcomed into the culture very fully by the people we came to know, though at first they were understandably suspicious of our motives. 'The Do-Gooders are coming' might have been the title of their song and with reason. We had to change our attitude however well intentioned it might have been.

After twelve years the time had come to leave. We were being asked to step forward into a wider world.

Chapter 3

A Bigger Picture

God is a beckoning word. He calls us out of ourselves and beyond ourselves, he is the God of surprises, always creating anew.[4]

I had been on a day's coach outing to Southend with a group from the Mayflower. We returned at 1.30 a.m. as the coach had broken down. I found David still up. He looked ashen. He invited me to sit down while he made some tea and told me that that day he had been to lunch with Mervyn Stockwood, the Bishop of Southwark. The Bishop had heard that David had married two people in a Baptist church in the diocese without asking permission and felt that he needed to give him a gentle rebuke.

This was true, but there was more. There was another agenda. The gentle rebuke was quickly delivered and then much to David's total surprise the Bishop had gone on to invite him to be his next suffragan, or assistant, as Bishop of Woolwich, following Bishop John Robinson who was retiring. His book *Honest to God* had caused major controversy in 1963 over its portrayal of the image of God. David asked for time to think.

He was still in shock and we talked. Nothing had been further from either of our minds. After twelve years, and needing a break to refresh, we had already planned to take a sabbatical leave in Scotland.

After some months of consultation and a good deal of secrecy to keep it out of the press, David accepted the Bishop's invitation. He was consecrated in Southwark Cathedral by the Archbishop of Canterbury, Michael Ramsey, on 11 June 1969, aged forty.

Jenny and I sat in the front row with Mrs Ramsey while I fought off panic attacks, hoping no one would notice. I was too proud to allow my condition to keep me at home that day, and Jenny needed me to be there.

The D'Oliveira affair

In the August of 1968 we took a hundred members of the May-flower to Belgium for a holiday. David came back after midnight one day, exhausted after dealing with an emergency when the hotel manager had given our party notice to quit the following day. Someone had been found smoking in bed. A reprieve had been negotiated, David using his halting French. On the midnight news I heard that D'Oliveira had not been picked for England to play South Africa. Calculating the risk of upsetting him, I broke the news to David. He was highly indignant, and left for London the following morning with little sleep, to research what was really behind the decision, and to confer with his colleagues. He discov-ered some disturbing facts. D'Oliveira had been born in South Africa where he was classified as 'coloured' under the apartheid regime – and banned from playing first-class cricket in his own country. He emigrated to England and became a British citizen. By 1966 D'Oliveira was being selected for the England team as an outstanding all-rounder and was an obvious choice for the Test side to play in South Africa in the 1968–69 series but he was not selected on apparently political and racial grounds.

David had been recalled to play for England in the Test side against South Africa and refused in protest at the omission of D'Oliveira. This set the cat among the Marylebone Cricket Club pigeons – the ruling elite of English cricket. At a specially called meeting of the MCC in Church House Westminster with regard to the D'Oliveira affair, David was accused of arrogance in using his position to embarrass the cricket authorities who felt under pres-sure with the publicity. It had recently been announced that he was to be the next Bishop of Woolwich. 'I don't know how the Bishop of Woolwich can wear his MCC tie!' called out someone disparag-ingly. A voice from the gallery replied, lightening the atmosphere, 'Down the back!' – a reference to his habitual clerical collar.

In protesting, David was in fact pursuing his Christian calling to act against injustice, which was now so clear and which demanded action, at whatever cost to himself. It might have been easier in some ways to sit tight and complain and protest in private. That way there would have been no risk; no rocking the boat and no change. But the D'Oliveira affair simply heightened David's right-eous indignation.

As a Test cricketer, and someone who was becoming a Christian leader, he felt called to stand by this excluded cricketer and, further, to join the fight with his friends in the anti-apartheid movement. He did not fall into the trap of doing this on his own, but took a lot of advice and sought support from people he trusted before going public. Desmond Tutu, who was to become Archbishop of Cape Town, and fellow cricketer Mike Brearley were among his most trusted friends and colleagues. In the end the MCC called off the South Africa tour. David lost one or two friendships over the D'Oliveira issue, which was painful and a cause of great sadness. Uncomfortable as it was at times, I supported him all the way.

When we were asked out to meals in those days, other guests often would pluck up the courage to question David and pin him down about his actions relating to race issues and also to unemployment or comprehensive education. This could happen at about a quarter to eleven at night when we were dropping with fatigue and ready to go home. Discussion would become embarrassingly heated at times. David would jokingly talk of writing his apology to the host before we arrived in future.

Becoming a bishop's family after life in an East London community was a radical change. Instead of sharing our lives with thirty people day and night, we now lived in a South London house in Peckham, attached to a Social Services Centre, opposite a newsagent, a comprehensive school and a pub. Instead of metal guards across our windows overlooking a scrap yard, and later a view of new post-war flats across the road, we had big clear windows, a modest garden and steps up to our front door.

After the relative intimacy of our Mayflower Family Centre life I did not at first find it easy to live with the new big-picture ministry. It felt draughty. Though we would often discuss the challenges David faced as a high-profile bishop, I would often act as devil's advocate, posing questions that the press might put to David in interviews. We would sometimes do this on long car journeys. He would always test his motives with a trusted friend or colleague. He rarely acted alone and without careful thought and briefing. I shared his beliefs totally, but at times feared for his reputation, and for ours as a family. I was conscious of the power of some elements of the more popular press to distort, as well as to inform, and sometimes to destroy. David was easy material because of his celebrity cricketing status, coupled with being a bishop of the Church of England. We had to accept that. But we also had a small daughter to consider.

At first it was lonely in Peckham, and I had to find ways of tackling that, as David was out most of the day and Jenny was now at school. Out of respect and apprehension, people tend to keep bishops and their wives at arm's length at first until they know them. They are on their best behaviour and afraid of being regarded as crawlers. It became necessary to make the first move to say hello if loneliness was to be kept at bay. I would sweep the steps some mornings and make friends with some of the children and passers-by. I found it helpful to join a local housing action group, unconnected with the Church, where I could connect with local people and be in touch with what concerned them most.

I was still battling with agoraphobia, but inching my way to more confidence. I shall always be grateful to two people who treated me normally at that time. One of them lived nearby and invited me to have lunch in her home. We became friends and would wash and dry our hair together, as she had an old-fashioned hairdryer with a hood, in her cellar. We would enjoy each other's company and share common interests. She made me feel that I had something to offer, despite my disability. She was and still is a good friend. Her home and friendship gave me a glimpse of heaven on earth and were major planks in building my house of confidence.

Gradually I found the confidence to drive to her house, which was another step towards recovery. By this time I was driving short distances in a Morris 1100 that a friend had given to me before she left the country. That generous gift played a huge part in my rehabilitation, as I felt safer in a car and had always enjoyed driving.

I was happy to entertain. David and I regularly invited people into our home for a buffet meal. We always looked forward to these occasions. Cooking held no fears for me and it was fun to meet a wide range of people: usually about fifteen at a time. One day though, I became puzzled as our room was filling up very quickly and seemed a bit more cramped than usual. David was late back from a meeting. I whispered my anxiety to him. He took

one look and said that we had next week's party here as well!
Thirty people now needed feeding instead of fifteen. I quickly
realised my mistake in putting the same date on the invitations to
both parties. I confessed to everyone and put people to work. It
was a rice dish. One opened a tin or two and another washed some
more lettuce; I cooked some more rice while another picked more
raspberries from the garden for the spare pavlova that I had put by.
I put the Archdeacon in charge of the coffee. It was one of the most
relaxed and happy evenings we ever spent.

Chapter 4

Our Liverpool Home

In my Liverpool home, In my Liverpool home
We speak with an accent exceedingly rare,
Meet under a statue exceedingly bare,
And if you want a Cathedral, we've got one to spare
In my Liverpool home.[5]

Six years living just off the Old Kent Road passed quickly. In the mid-1970s, press speculation began when it became clear that Stuart Blanch was leaving Liverpool, as its bishop, to become the Archbishop of York. David's name was being suggested as Stuart's successor, together with the names of others. To me in my ignorance, Liverpool seemed a long way away. We decided not even to discuss the issue until reality dawned. We were very content where we were. Then while we were on a break looking after David's mother who was recovering from a hip operation, speculation changed to reality. The telephone rang. It was David's secretary saying, 'I think it's come. Shall I open it?' The envelope within an envelope was opened and the mystery dissolved.

We moved to Liverpool in 1975. We had not been allowed to see the house beforehand, but were sent photographs. It was a Victorian merchant's house which lay up a winding drive, in a suburb of Liverpool, had eight bedrooms and a garden of nearly two acres on a hillside. There were just three of us to make a home there. We arrived to bare boards, but there was a good atmosphere to the place and we grew to love it.

Soon after the move someone asked me if I was lonely. 'Oh no!' I replied, a little too quickly. In fact I knew only three people in Liverpool and wondered how I was going to adjust and belong to this new city. Those three friends became my lifeline when I was very lonely and too proud to admit it. It took three years before I felt I belonged. Then there was no holding me. I fell in love with the place.

From the beginning I set about cooking in order to fill the house with delicious smells. I put on my favourite music to fill it with good sounds. The garden had suffered neglect in the interregnum and presented a challenge. I loved it, and revelled in the challenge to create something that all could enjoy. By then Jenny was thirteen and attending a local comprehensive school and had her own settling in to do which was not easy for her.

David put his heart and soul into his work. I put mine into making a warm and welcoming home for him and Jenny to return to, a home in which he could both work in peace and relax, and she could entertain her friends.

The diocesan diary took over and David was swept into the life of a diocesan bishop. We put our minds to hospitality. I was a mother, housekeeper and cook for the stream of guests, including David's regular staff meetings which took place in the house. We entertained a great many people and the house and garden were used for many events down the years.

I became involved with the Family Service Unit in Liverpool. There were also expectations that I would provide a programme and support for the wives of clergy in the diocese, and organise a conference for them.

In the cathedral I was expected to sit in the front row and found this daunting as I still suffered panic attacks and did not want to make a fuss. Few people knew about these, as I was doing my fidgeting under a cloak bought specially to hide it, and hoping that the anxiety would go away one day soon. My problems became public after agreeing to participate in the *Anno Domini* programme on BBC TV looking at David's move to Liverpool as its bishop. The sensitivity and integrity of Bill Nicholson, the producer, persuaded me that it would help many viewers if I was willing to share my vulnerability. He even prepared two reels, one with my interview and one without, saying that all I had to do was to ring half an hour before the programme went out if I wanted to withdraw. With that support and understanding, I decided to go for it. We had over a thousand letters from viewers expressing relief and gratitude, saying they did not feel alone after hearing us. For myself, it was a key turning point in my recovery. I began to come out of hiding and did not have to live a double life any more. A letter from Bill Nicholson, who later wrote the play *Shadowlands*, quoted the words from St John's Gospel, 'You shall know the truth and the truth shall make you free.' And so it proved, eventually.

Meanwhile I revelled in the music of the cathedral under the leadership of the organist Professor Ian Tracey. I sang in a number of the choirs that rehearsed and performed in that awesome building. The vergers became my friends. Also I was always made to feel part of the family at the Metropolitan Cathedral, or Paddy's Wigwam as it is affectionately called locally, at the other end of Hope Street.

It had been exhausting living two lives: smiling on the outside and quaking on the inside. But I had found a way of coping which took me through each day. In fact it took seven years before I acknowledged that I could not heal myself, and went for help. Up until then I still hoped that the problem would go away by itself, and I did not relish the idea of consulting a psychologist. But I became increasingly conscious that the vibrant city of Liverpool was like a perpetual party, and I felt on the edge, like a wallflower. My gift of life was being wasted. I wanted to join in. So it became blindingly clear one day that I could not cure myself and would need outside help. With bated breath I burnt my boats and made an appointment with a clinical psychologist outside Liverpool.

For three years I paid regular visits to her. I came to trust her. With great skill she teased out of me some of the experiences which appeared to have broken down my self-confidence and set up such crippling fears. I felt she believed in me. Crucially she helped me to rediscover my inner authority and my ability to make decisions. 'You are a free agent,' she would say. That meant learning to set out options and then choosing which way I wanted to go. She helped me to re-engage with my will, my life force, and to use it without feeling that 'I want to' was always selfish.

For example, one day with difficulty I told her that I was fearful of travelling on the Underground. 'Why?' she asked. 'Because I am frightened that I might fall on to the live rail involuntarily.' She said, 'Do you want to?' 'Goodness no!' I exclaimed. 'Then you won't,' she said with authority. I believed her. I was released from that fear for ever. Twenty years later I can travel happily on the Underground and thank God for this person and for the turning point towards the full recovery I have made. David knew of my battle, but never pushed me or ceased to believe that I would pull through eventually. Belief is a potent instrument of healing; the knowledge that someone not only loves you, but also believes in your ability to make effective decisions.

At the heart of it all was our chapel. Here was a quiet space half way up the stairs in Bishop's Lodge, curtained off from a meeting room. Just four of us met each morning before work to say Morning Prayer. We sat informally in a semi-circle; the bishop's chaplain, George the gardener, David and me. We kept it simple. There was a plain wooden cross on the hessian-covered wall and we lit a candle. Guests would join us if they wished. Each of us took it in turns to lead the prayers. Afterwards we would discuss the day ahead for a few minutes, raising any questions or problems. In this way we kept in touch and in tune with each other on a daily basis. We were also conscious of being part of the wider Church. Together we touched base with our Maker.

It became a most important time for each of us as individuals, and as a team. It earthed us, and at the same time lifted our sights above our day-to-day work. Here we experienced a rare intimacy while maintaining our differing roles. It was a time and place for stillness and for acknowledging God in an attitude of worship together for half an hour before work. It became the bedrock. For me it helped to form a habit of being comfortable with stillness in an active life. It created a place that could be revisited again and again, even for a minute, during busy and stressful times. The nineteenth-century missionary Amy Carmichael wrote: 'Hast thou one minute? Then hem it with quietness.'[6]

Now and again there were invitations for David to represent the Liverpool Diocese further afield and to visit churches abroad. In 1989 the church leaders of South Africa invited David and his colleague and friend, the Roman Catholic Archbishop of Liverpool Derek Worlock, to visit them. The two bishops were invited to come to listen, and to encourage the churches, during the state of emergency that had been declared by President Botha in 1985. Nelson Mandela was still in prison.

I was invited to join them, together with Julian Filochowski who was head of CAFOD[7] at the time, and Derek's chaplain, John Furnival, and the invitation was accepted. In South Africa we stayed in people's homes, ate with them, played with their children and enjoyed their company.

Very poor people, rich in kindness and living in shacks, under a blanket of smoke, showed a generosity and a dignity that took our breath away. Marginalised in Soweto, they were hungry for visitors. They showed this in their smiles, their posture, their songs and dancing, their hospitality and their gifts.

On the only occasion when the press accompanied us, there were filmed interviews with the two bishops. As I was not needed, I called on a woman in her home. She lived in a shack with her family. I was assured that I would be told when the main party moved on. Unfortunately they forgot and moved on without telling me. I was left alone in the township with no knowledge of where to go next.

It was a moment of truth. I had found a friend in this woman. Now I could either panic and struggle on alone and embarrassed, feeling alienated, or treat the people as my friends, as I needed their help. I opted for the latter. After all I was publishing my first book[8] that autumn on facing fear and finding courage and needed to practise what I was writing. It was the final test.

For a long moment I struggled with deep-rooted prejudice. In front of me stood four men who had been keeping an eye on things and had seen what was going on. I was ashamed that I even doubted their goodness because I was afraid of robbery or rape. I cast those thoughts from my head and heart into the sand at my feet and stepped forward to meet them. My fear evaporated. At that moment my agoraphobia withered and died. If John Bunyan had written my story he would have created a new person whose name changed from Mrs Fear-All to Mrs Love-your-Neighbour; or from Mrs Mistrust to Mrs Trust-and-be-Thankful. She would have looked Master Don't-Trust-a-Soul in the eyes and he would have slunk away into the shadows.

The four men stood waiting and I made signs to describe my predicament. They quickly understood. They were not suspicious of me and showed me the way. I walked through lines of shacks, unafraid and totally in the hands of my hosts, thanking them as I went. Eventually I spotted the others in the distance. I joined the official party, surrounded with laughing playing children. Within the space of half an hour I had crossed the Rubicon. But I was brought down to earth by hearing that no one had missed me! That day I waved farewell to the dreaded panic attacks for ever. The following month, at the time of publication, I had to step into the public arena in my own right.

Africa changes you. Poor people are rich in generosity. When visiting Nigeria on an earlier occasion we travelled with three pieces of luggage between us. We returned with thirteen. Pictures, carvings and cloth were showered on us. The gift that made the deepest impression was the infectious joy. This and their welcome, despite the poverty, made us look again at our values and question them. In the Nigerian villages, we noted that the children could play outside their homes safely. They were everyone's responsibility. We were told that if a child showed exceptional academic promise, then the village would come together and fundraise to give that child the opportunity for further education. African people have much to teach us about belonging and interdependence, about community and the value of education.

It is always a tragedy to hear of someone who has been found dead days or weeks later in their own home. We have much to learn from Africa and its people who keep an eye on each other. Poverty throws people together. There is a need to review our culture and notice those who have no family or friends, and who are being pushed to the edges of society by the affluence and greed of others. We can come near to them. They have something to give us: something that we lack and need, and something that will not perish. They are our friends in waiting.

Liverpool has a way of ensnaring heart and soul. It is a vibrant city with a spectacular waterfront, and its people are known for their friendliness and humour. We laughed and wept together. We stayed up till past one in the morning as our comedian Ken Dodd had us aching with laughter. We swelled with proper pride at wonders of the International Garden Festival in 1984. This was also the year that David's mother died. In 1989 we grieved at the devastating loss of 96 football fans at the Hillsborough disaster.

Every Sunday, David and I visited a different parish church. We were welcomed into countless homes and organisations in diocese and city. We shared the pain of the Toxteth riots in 1981, which erupted as a result of long-standing tension between the police and the black community.

The two cathedrals at either end of Hope Street saw history made when Pope John Paul visited Liverpool in 1982. Sister Antony and her embroidery team stitched a large banner depicting the occasion of the visit and included David among the clergy worked into the piece. Half-way along the street now, almost opposite the Philharmonic Hall, is a sculpture to commemorate the ecumenical friendship and contribution that David and Derek Worlock made during their years in the city. It was unveiled by the Mayor on 23 May 2008. It depicts two slim set-apart, fourteen-feet-high open doors in bronze, with a life-sized representation of each man walking, and robed. On the back of each door there are bas-relief panels depicting aspects of their lives and work. At David's feet there is a cricket ball. This statue was the initiative of the city's evening newspaper, the *Liverpool Echo*, and was largely funded by local people. It was skilfully and imaginatively crafted by Stephen Broadbent.

In 1997, after twenty-two years in Liverpool, David was sixty-eight. He felt that he had given all he could and decided to retire. This was a big step for us both, after being in the public eye throughout our life together. Our years in Liverpool were fulfilling and deeply happy. There is something about the city that melts the heart of the stiffest Southerner.

We began the gargantuan task of reducing and packing up twenty-two years of gathered possessions, and of saying good-bye to our friends and colleagues in the church and city we had come to love. This would be a major bereavement, but rather than concentrate on the loss we looked forward to a new life together. Jenny married Donald Sinclair in 1988. We looked forward to spending more time with them too.

I was thrilled at the prospect of being private and having more time together despite the warnings of some who said, 'He'll be under your feet all day!' I thought that was unlikely, as we had designed our marriage to include spaces in our togetherness, as Kahlil Gibran advocated in his meditation on marriage:

> Sing and Dance together and be joyous, but let each one of you be alone.
> ...
> And stand together, yet not too near together.[9]

There is a place for learning to be comfortable alone. The wisdom of Gibran was to prove invaluable later on when I was to face the biggest challenge of my life.

Chapter 5

Retirement Idyll

… stand together, yet not too near together.

We left Liverpool in a cascade of multi-coloured balloons and glorious music. The Farewell Service contained a high note of thanksgiving for David's ministry. Mark Boyling, then the Precentor, had designed an imaginative liturgy. This included an opportunity for us both to walk around the packed cathedral and bid a personal farewell to individuals, representatives of parishes and organisations in an orderly fashion. This was within the setting of eucharistic worship. It was a poignant and moving occasion as twenty-two momentous years in Liverpool Diocese swam before our eyes. We had become adopted 'scousers' – as Liverpool people are affectionately known.

The balloons were released from the rafters of the cathedral as we departed. They helped us all to smile through the mixed emotions. It was a wonderful way to go.

We walked out into the night. Outside it was a dark September evening. George, our driver, was waiting with the car. Someone had tied more balloons to the back bumper which bore the words, 'You're never too old to party.' We took this to mean that we could throw our hats into the air and start to relax.

David removed his cope and mitre, and, in the car headlights, we waved good-bye to the bystanders. We climbed into the back of the car. David was still in his purple cassock and white rochet, looking to an outsider like someone in fancy dress. We drove off feeling like a wedding couple with the balloons fluttering behind. In a few minutes a police car drew up and indicated to us to stop. They had a few words with George, asking him to remove the balloons as they were obscuring the registration plate. An officer peered through the back window, looking rather bemusedly at

David. He said: 'It is all right this time, sir. But please never do this again.' 'I promise', said David with the suspicion of a smile, 'that I will never do this again.' We drove on into retirement.

So began a deeply happy few years together when for the first time we became relatively private people. We had prepared carefully.

Some people dread retirement because it feels like a step towards dying and death; the loss of identity and of meaning. This is especially true for those who have no hobby or outside interest and who have sunk themselves totally into their job for a lifetime. Retirement can be a bereavement in itself with the loss of role and of colleagues; loss of the cut and thrust of belonging to the working world. It makes all the difference to prepare for the day of retirement and to allow a dream or two to surface of what retirement could be.

Much as I loved our working life in Liverpool, I could not wait to create a new life with David where we could relax together more privately, as ordinary people with neighbours and interests, and without the diocesan diary taking precedence. We had our dreams.

We had discussed the future long and hard, making lists and agreeing what each wanted in retirement. We both wanted a garden. I wanted a community to belong to again and I wanted to be near water. David wanted access to a city. As our families and friends were scattered from London, Dorset and Sussex, to Ireland, and later to Scotland, we had decided to stay north-west.

Our new house was detached with a garden, in a road alongside others, and by the River Dee. We faced the Welsh hills. We had our backs to Liverpool and were now in the Chester Diocese. We had often slipped under the river through the Mersey tunnel on our days off to relax in this place and walk by the river. But we knew only a handful of people this side of the water.

The day we were given the keys to our new house in September 1997 was one of the most exciting in my life. It felt like being married for the first time. It was forty years on from our challenging beginning. We were older and ready for change. They were keys to much more than the house. They were keys to a new kind of freedom and to a new life.

The generosity of our vendors made a huge difference to the transition. Despite the fact that they were moving to Wales, they reached out to us by throwing a lunch party to enable us to meet the neighbours, and for them to meet us. About fifteen people came. It was a great success. We agreed to exchange keys with those who would be our nearest neighbours. We felt among friends and trusted one another. Years later, hardly a week goes by without someone expressing how fortunate they feel to live in such a friendly road.

Though tired from nearly a year of farewells and dealing with the clutter of two decades, and the upheaval of the move itself, both of us were healthy and looked forward to some more relaxing years together. It felt good to be free to design our own shared space and time. We decided to spend the first six months with a virtually empty diary to get the feel of the new life, to develop a new rhythm and to gather ideas of what each wanted to do.

We had exchanged the majestic listed beeches in Bishop's Lodge garden for the wide skies and tidal waters of the Dee Estuary. We had neighbours. Once again after over thirty years of being in tied bishops' houses, we were in a community, but we had our own private front door. We had no definable roles now except that of retired bishop and wife. We stepped into a cloud of unknowing, but full of hopes and dreams and with a spirit of adventure. That spirit never left us.

Retirement could have been quite difficult, particularly for David. But he had been ready to leave Liverpool, and felt he had completed what he could give, even though he would miss his colleagues. I was ready for different reasons; not least because we would have time together, and hopefully for me there would be more opportunity to pursue my own interests and hobbies. For both of us, however, there was at last the chance to design our own lives as husband and wife with the freedom to choose. It was as though we were visiting this place of being alone together in our marriage for the first time, since our traumatic post-honeymoon beginnings all those years ago.

Nearby was a railway station which enabled passengers to get to London and Liverpool easily. But we resolved to look forward and not to visit Liverpool, except to catch a train, for at least three years, in order to give some space to David's successor, when appointed. Instead we looked to Wales and Chester for our cultural pursuits of theatre and music. We cut our moorings. David had resigned from all his Liverpool commitments, and so had I.

The years that followed were deeply happy. As time passed it warmed my heart to hear David say often, 'I do love this place.' He set up a small study upstairs with his books where he spent most mornings. He took a bus each week to Wirral Metropolitan College where he had signed up for a ten-week computer course.

After forty years of having a secretary to help deal with his heavy mail, David now dealt alone with his considerable correspondence. He did it with flair, and increasing confidence, and even with enjoyment. Later he wrote his autobiography, using his computing and word-processing skills.

David was welcomed by the Bishop of Chester who gave him a role in the diocese as an assistant bishop, so his priesthood continued to be exercised, which he found fulfilling. Sometimes he presided and preached at our local church, which gave us a deep and gentle welcome. But usually we sat at the back, which enabled us to settle gradually into being regular parishioners instead of visiting a new church every Sunday, as we had done for nearly thirty years.

When invitations came in to take on time-consuming commitments he was keen to point out that he was a *retired* bishop. We both enjoyed our neighbours, with time to chat 'over the fence'. Together we planned our garden. David could watch cricket at his leisure.

Just before Christmas 1997 I was called to do jury service in Liverpool. This lasted for a few weeks and was another new experience. David welcomed me home each day with a meal. Life could not get much better. He had become a proficient cook specialising in soups. To my delight, he took a full share in the domestic round which gave me a new liberation, opening up fresh areas of choice and the possibility of writing again.

David loved to walk by the River Dee each morning before breakfast. We both painted a little and enjoyed visiting theatres and attending concerts. We also enjoyed having friends round for a meal. It was like being married for the first time, though with much of our life behind us as well as in front.

Although we had plenty of hobbies, we also realised that we would need to step out into the community if we wanted to find new friends, so we joined a choir. I had always belonged to one, but David had not sung in a choir since being lead treble in his school choir, singing in Sherborne Abbey. In the St Peter's Singers we made a new set of friends and enjoyed the music, performing in a concert twice a year.

We both found the garden a place of refreshment as well as a challenge to put in the necessary work. Not only was a new home of our own among the joys, we had a garden which needed attention. Little did I know then what a friend that was to become. The garden was a shared love. The space was there waiting for a design.

The people of Liverpool Diocese had given us a generous cheque on our retirement, and others had given us garden vouchers. This gave us a wonderful freedom to plan. After nine months of sketches, poring over garden books, sharing ideas and making decisions we began staking out the new shape in the snow. We felt that we needed to design something that would still be possible for us to manage when we reached our eighties.

Now it has matured and it has ministered to us in different ways. It became part of us. It called us out to breathe the scented air when we were weary. There was music too as the birds sang their hearts out in the early morning and evening. Flowers provided colour and scent, and instant gifts for friends. Fruit included apples and figs, redcurrants and gooseberries; and digging new potatoes still fills me with the thrill of a child discovering buried treasure. We ate and drank al fresco with friends and family.

The garden cajoled and called us. It comforted and cheered us when we needed it. It entertained and nourished us. It also thrilled us, like the day when a wisteria, a gift from friends, flowered for the first time after several years. It was always there for us, full of living and dying and moving on. Yet as with friendship of any kind it needed patience, time and effort for the relationship to thrive.

David continued to walk each morning before breakfast on the sandy beach among clam shells and to the sound of curlews and dunlin. We sat up in bed each day to a view of the Welsh hills and the ebbing and flowing of the Dee Estuary. There was a remarkable luminosity in the air, which was a gift for painters. This was as near to Paradise as you could get.

David found he enjoyed preparing sermons as never before. Instead of being expected to speak on several occasions in a week, now he could start thinking about his talk at the beginning of the week before the following Sunday. We both enjoyed painting. We holidayed in a self-catering flat high over the coast in Aberdyfi in West Wales. There we could paint, read and walk on the beach under the wide skies to our heart's content.

Six months flew by. We had both begun to accept speaking engagements again. Hodder Headline wanted David to publish his autobiography. Darton, Longman and Todd had given me an open invitation to produce another book. David always encouraged me to write.

To crown it all, we heard that we were to become grandparents. Several months after we retired, in September 1998, Stuart was born. His brother Gilles arrived just under two years later. What joy has followed.

Chapter 6

Unwelcome News

He who can say, 'In the end, God,' has a strength that is impossible to fathom.[10]

Stuart was baptised in London. My parents were now living together in a retirement home where they were well cared for. My father travelled by train from Dorset to London, on his eighty-ninth birthday, to share in this special family time. We waved to him and my sister Evelyn as they left Waterloo station to return home. We could not have known that in three weeks he would be with us no more. My father died in his chair, dressed and ready for church on Advent Sunday. In his hand was a note to the local mayor who was a friend, with a word of encouragement. This was his last act. He died as he lived: an encourager. This was a big shock for my mother who needed nursing care and was in the same room when he died. The news stunned us all. It was a devastating loss for me as I loved my father dearly. I was the eldest sibling and therefore felt some responsibility for setting the tone of our mourning. Tears were not to be hidden or despised. We needed to be close to our mother.

The morning after my father's death, my sister and I visited her in their retirement home. This was new country for us. We were treading new ground. To our consternation, my father's bed had already been removed and my mother's bed had been placed in a new position the other side of the room. The remaining furniture in the room had been moved round and my mother was looking dazed. Two people, each with a machine, were vacuuming the carpet. It was noisy and busy and it could only be described as a rumpus. In my indignation, I called over the noise of the vacuum cleaners, 'Mum, this is your room. You don't have to move your bed!' Her reply was typically practical and without thought for herself. 'They have to get on,' she said. Perhaps the truth had not yet dawned on her. Perhaps she was better prepared than we were. They had been married for sixty-four years. Maybe it was my sister and I who had the problem. We sat quietly with my mother, over a cup of tea, absorbing the shock of knowing that Dad was not coming back.

The family came from all directions to help prepare for the funeral. We were to witness the love that people had locally, and further afield, for my father, and for my mother too. This was a joy and an inspiration to us. We found strength in each other and in our different gifts. The local priest was deeply supportive, sensitive and helpful as she sat at her computer, listening to our wishes, and tweaking the liturgy to suit us. She was ready with suggestions without being domineering.

My father had prepared for his death carefully. He had left model instructions and copied them to my brother, my sisters and me, which made our job easier. The instructions were practical, with telephone numbers and details of whom to contact. They were sensitive and left us free to plan but with suggestions for the service that did not bind us. This thoughtful preparation gave us a lead, but also freed us to mourn together and share our memories unhurriedly. David was asked to preach. For me the family was a strong and loving unit of practical support. We also were not afraid to laugh when recalling moments of our father's life. He laughed easily. His legacy of laughter had already begun, as I was very soon to find out.

For me the practical side of death and dying had remained a mystery until my father died. Some of us grow up rather late and I had not seen a dead body till this moment. I decided to remove the 'block'. I loved my father and felt it was the time to do this. Very apprehensively, I took a deep breath and, together with David, went into the Chapel of Rest to see his body. It was an odd experience. I was glad that David was there. Although it was clearly my father's face, there was something not quite right about his appearance. I tried not to think too much about the padding and tinting that takes place to present a likeness after death. I wept a little and found myself talking naturally to his remains, and saying thank you for so much. Then we left. The 'block' had shifted. I had more than survived the experience. Facing the reality reduced the fear. But there was still a question stirring in my mind.

Once outside the Chapel of Rest, the penny dropped. It became clear what had been amiss. My father often saw the funny side of life. I returned to the chapel, alone this time, and asked him what the joke was. In a flash I saw it. We had not been invited to dress his body in his ordinary clothes by the funeral director. In our ignorance we had not thought to ask if we could. Ordinary clothes would have included a tweed jacket from the Oxfam shop and a shirt, a jumper and trousers, and his rimless glasses. Instead he was decked in white satin frills right up to his neck, and without his glasses. I had my answer to what was wrong and came out of the chapel chuckling – I think my father must have been chuckling too. We saw no need to disturb things further and left him peacefully in his frills.

After the funeral, my mother sat outside in the churchyard in her wheelchair, greeting people. She was wrapped up for a cold December day and buoyed up by seeing so many old friends. They made all the difference at such a time. My father had requested no plaque or memorial. His ashes lie in the churchyard of Holy Trinity, Bradpole in Dorset, under the grass. We planted some snowdrops close by in gentle defiance of his wishes.

Losing my father so early in our retirement was a blow. But there were some shock absorbers which made a pathway for joy to do its work. They came in various guises. The love of family and friends came first on the list; also a sense of humour – bequeathed by my father. The prayers of the local church fellowship were palpably uplifting. The writing of a daily journal helped me to sort out my feelings through logging day-to-day events; certain pieces of music brought peace and real comfort. The garden too was a key place of healing and joy. These, and other shock absorbers, prevented the family feeling that we were alone. We knew that there were others in the wings should we stumble and fall; others who would be there calmly when we needed to shed tears. There was life after a death.

But by his example my father had helped us all to accept the inevitable. David and I returned to our new home and garden resolved to pick up our life again and make the most of our time together.

My mother

My mother remained in the retirement home in Dorset, near one of my sisters. But by the end of the year, there were signs that the home was struggling to survive. Mum would have to be moved. The home eventually closed days before Christmas 2000. We had to act quickly to save her unnecessary trauma. That Christmas was a nightmare. We both had coughs and flu. One of David's teeth broke. The phone was hot with calls to and from my sisters and brother discussing what to do for my mother and making appointments to visit local nursing homes just in case. On 27 December, she and we decided that she should come to be near me. During this time two faithful friends came to be with David and me and to help us along.

My brother and two sisters had taken responsibility for caring for my mother during her declining years. Now it was my turn. I had visited eleven places for a suitable nursing home near us with a vacancy. Only days before the closure of Mum's retirement home one became available. On 11 January 2001, my two sisters drove my mother up the motorway from Dorset to the Wirral. We all went with her to the nursing home and settled her in comfortably with some of her own things. She took the move well. The window of her room looked across the sands of West Kirby on the Wirral where she and my father had met serving on a beach mission in 1919 as teenagers. It was their second meeting and they had fallen in love. Her life was now turning full circle.

For David and me her move to the Wirral naturally meant a change in our pattern of life in order to include regular visits, and outings, for an 89-year-old who needed a good deal of care. For the next two years, until her death, we visited my mother regularly, reading aloud and playing some of her favourite music on CD.

Local friends were particularly kind. One sent flowers and another read aloud to her each week. One of the abiding images of my mother in those years was when we opened the door to her room. From her bed, she would fling her arms wide open in welcome and gladness that we had come. I have always felt this to be a foretaste of the kind of greeting we may expect in heaven.

This was the person who had shown such courage throughout her life, battling against many odds, including asthma. She loved her Bible and had taught me to pray to a God whom we could call a friend. She had brought up three of us during the Second World War while doodlebugs flew overhead. My youngest sister came along later. This was the woman who would walk five miles to the nearest shops and back, with two toddlers. This was the woman who knitted complicated Fair Isle jumpers from recycled wool and without a pattern. She painted, and played the piano well, including a party piece played all on the black notes, called 'In Cheerful Mood', which we all loved. My mother showed us how to keep an open home where all were welcome, whether there was anything in the larder or not.

She was now on her last lap. Death and life were continuing to be close companions. Moving on and letting go is in the rhythm of life and it helps if we're ready, knowing that God is there around every corner, beckoning us on. All we have to do is to follow. That, at least, is the theory. For my mother this was a long haul. For us this was both a privilege and a learning curve in learning to wait with her with loving patience for her release. At least she was not in pain, but weary and ready to go.

Chapter 7

The Shock and the Shock Absorbers

Let me use disappointment as material for patience …
Let me use suspense as material for perseverance.[11]

Early in our retirement David had been honoured with a peerage. This introduced a new dimension for him. He made regular visits to London to attend the House of Lords, which enabled him to play a part in the bigger picture again and to meet up with friends and former colleagues in the city. It also meant he could see more of his grandsons in London. Occasionally I would join him. He always came back stimulated and fulfilled, and also glad to be home. While I was pleased for David, I missed him at first and felt I was losing him to the old work pattern after such a new and idyllic beginning. Once again the diary threatened spontaneity. It meant another adjustment. He was only away three days a fortnight and I soon found the time flying. Nevertheless it was a foretaste of bereavement, a taste of what was to come. Meanwhile I was learning a little more about caring through visiting my mother.

The times of regular separation in fact proved invaluable to us both for differing reasons. We had studied in our marriage to leave space for each to breathe and to grow, but we were close. For me, David's journeys to London were a good preparation for what was to follow. For him, these visits meant intellectual stimulation and a feeling of being regularly in the mainstream again.

There was a cloud on the horizon. David had complained of pain in his abdomen and he was getting dizzy spells. After a couple of weeks he reluctantly made an appointment to see the doctor. There were tests and eventually the results came through. Something was wrong. He was referred to a consultant. Pressure was building up. He saw the consultant alone, and, while feeling desperately anxious, I could see he was preoccupied and needed time to think before telling me of the outcome. I did not wish to urge him to disclose his news till he was ready. I think we were both holding our breath. Two long days later he told me that it might be cancer.

So that was it. But 'might be' is not the same as 'is'. This gave a tiny fanlight of hope. But doubt is a disturbing bedfellow. We would have to sleep with it. There would have to be more tests before we could be sure. The same day that David gave me the news we attended the funeral of a civic colleague who had tragically committed suicide. It was a difficult day.

I struggled privately with divided loyalties. There was an element of shock to handle despite the question mark over David's diagnosis. How was I going to cope with the practical implications of being a grandmother to my grandsons, a daughter to my mother and a wife to my husband? Who should come first?

I was under the doctor for a throat problem and went to see him. I shared our news with him and my dilemma. The doctor was in no doubt as to my priority. This released a lot of the built-up tension of recent weeks. I left the surgery knowing that David was to be my first priority, whatever happened.

Shocks and surprises are distinct from one another. The Jesuit Gerard Hughes has written that God is a 'God of Surprises, and God is in the surprises'. He is there in the shocks, too, if we look for him.

Sometimes we are taken off guard especially when life is going smoothly; when we are so wrapped up in our own happiness that we forget for a while that bad news such as sudden death is part of many people's lives. If we do not prepare for these times and are not ready to face them squarely when things are going well, we shall be rocked off balance by them. We will find ourselves crying out, 'It's not fair!' or 'Why me?' or 'God, where are you?' There is nothing wrong in being shocked. But shock needs handling. Our little boat needed steadying.

Christ's way of dealing with death and dying is a model of how to cope. He talked about death over a meal with his friends. He even shouted at God as he was dying! 'My God! Why have you forsaken me?' For a Christian it is about friendship with God, with each other and with ourselves. Keeping the connection with God is vital – even if we have to shout at him! Christ showed us how to do this through his words on the cross.

We awaited the results of further tests on David. Our retirement idyll had received a body blow. But nothing could take away the joy of those first few years.

The consultant broke the news gently but firmly when she told us that it was probably cancer. She was a rock and continued to remain one. Surgery was offered quickly. David was due to take part in the Thanksgiving Service in Westminster Abbey for the life of his good friend and fellow Test cricketer Colin Cowdrey. This was to take place at the end of March 2001 – in a fortnight. He decided to wait until after the service to submit to the scalpel. We held on to our secret. He was still having dizzy spells and had fainted during some rather daunting X-rays.

The day after the visit to the consultant, he was in great form. Like facing the fast bowling of the Australian Keith Miller, he drove the news to the boundary. His first reaction was to say, 'Let's get on with it. I've got to die of something!' I could only applaud his pugnacity. Hearing the 'die' word on his lips was a bit of a jolt, but naming it somehow neutralised the deadening effect of simply keeping it in the imagination. His positive reaction would set the tone for all of us in the days ahead. I was feeling relatively at peace, though I suspect there was an element of unreality and disbelief.

We decided on a strategy to share the news. We would first tell close family and some special friends. We also told our bishop, Peter Forster, of Chester. Sharing our burden like this was a relief and we began to relax. Jenny heard the news first. This was a terrible blow for her, and also for David's sister, Mary. Jenny immediately and wisely suggested I told a local friend.

I rang a person I felt I could trust to sit still with me and asked if she had half an hour to spare as I thought I might need to shed some tears. She and her husband dropped everything and I went straight round. They were the perfect shock absorbers. This took a friendship to a deeper level and one which has sustained me ever since. I returned home ready for the next stage.

We received a wonderful note from another friend and neighbour which said:

Bother!
Should be OK for the cricket season.
Can we be temporary assistant gardeners
and mowers of lawn?
Thank you for sharing with us.
Much love from us both ... keep in touch.
Good excuse for some smart pyjamas.

Notes like this say everything that needs to be said. The words resonated with Christ's own words, 'I will never leave you nor forsake you.' Being there for one another is part of God's spirit in action. God is friendship.

Then came the question of whether or not to inform the press. News was bound to get out, and might be exaggerated. Cancer still spelt death for many, and we were keen to prevent any suggestion that David was imminently dying. With his agreement, I rang the Chester Diocesan Press Officer, with a simple statement of fact for their information. We wanted positive news to filter out, but it needed to be factual and brief without being sensational. He entered into our situation with the compassion of a good priest and the astute thinking of an able professional pressman.

The news was out and from then onwards there was to be no hiding place and no going back. We quickly began to realise that a hiding place is not the place to be if you want to experience the love that people are waiting to offer. Love is the best shock absorber of all. Riding the tidal wave of people's loving concern, however, needed grace and energy: grace to receive and energy to acknowledge seriously the many practical offers of help and then to weave them into our lives. We found ourselves woven into a tapestry of kindness.

Gradually we felt free to talk about David's condition more widely as and when it felt natural to do so. I plunged into the chocolate biscuit tin for comfort. The Macmillan Cancer Care nurse assigned to us visited our home where we had an unhurried conversation. We were reassured and impressed by her attention to both patient and carer, and by her ability to listen and to understand our particular needs. She helped us to face the facts. Outside it was snowing. Foot and Mouth disease was taking hold of cattle in many parts of the country. The clocks had gone forward and Cambridge won the Oxford and Cambridge boat race. Spring was round the corner and this made our problems easier to face. It would have been so much harder in the depths of winter.

On our way to London for the service for Colin Cowdrey, I suggested gently that we might raise some of the difficult questions and discuss them on the way back in the train. The 'What if?' questions lurked beneath the surface. They were tapping on the door and needed an airing. David agreed to think about this. His dizziness came and went and the pain and discomfort continued. He took part in the service and all was well.

There was a difficult moment for me as I entered the Abbey. I had taken care to ask advice about the dress code and was encouraged to wear something as bright as possible. The family wanted a note of thanksgiving to be struck and would not be wearing black themselves. So I wore a deep red dress and jacket.

Leaving David to robe in the vestry, I was conducted down the aisle of the Abbey in front of hundreds. A seat had been reserved for me among the peers and peeresses. Baroness Young was next to me and John and Norma Major were behind. Ronnie Corbett and his wife were in front. To my acute embarrassment, they were all in black except Norma Major and me. I suspect my face matched my suit. I was not into making fashion statements and on occasions like this I had wanted to fit in. But I have a mind that sees cartoons emerging, so eventually I saw the funny side! Nevertheless I resolved from that moment never again to attend a funeral or service of thanksgiving in anything but black. I only broke the resolution once, four years later, at David's own Thanksgiving Service.

On the way back on the train we had the important conversation about the difficult questions of death and dying. The 'What if you died?' was one of the most difficult, and 'How will you cope when I am gone?' was another. The conversation meant that all was now open between us and we became less afraid to face facts as they emerged.

That night in my diary I wrote, 'God bless my loved one. I want him back.' As I had survived cancer all those years ago, it seemed reasonable to hope that he would too. We would fight the disease together. We both felt underpinned by people's prayers and by the medical care. The struggle would be shared. We were not alone.

The evening before David's operation, we attended the healing service in our local church. We both went forward for the laying on of hands.

Chapter 8

Soul Friends

O the comfort, the inexpressible comfort, of feeling safe with a person neither having to weigh thought or measure words, but only to pour them right out, just as they are – chaff and grain together – knowing that a faithful hand will take and sift them, then, with a breath of kindness blow the rest away.[12]

For some years in my private devotions I had been using a book of personal prayers and meditations for every day by Ruth Etchells. This had become a remarkable aid to my faith. The author, a respected theologian, has a gift not only for the English language, but also for transmitting her personal understanding and experience of God in a most accessible way. She enables the reader to think of being an adventurer, and that God is there in the unknown. Each new adventure in life can be regarded as 'a new territory of grace'.[13] This struck a chord with me and became a stepping stone to looking for God in the waves of confusion as they threatened to wash over us. Cancer attacks the body but not the soul. He would be there somewhere. We only had to look for him in order to find a safe and stable way of moving into new territory.

David came through the operation for a bowel resection well. I visited him in the High Dependency Unit where he was in good spirits. His first words to me were, 'I love you. I'm so pleased you're here. You're healing me.' What a treat for me to hear those words at such a time, even though it may have been partly the morphine talking! He left the High Dependency Unit without any tubes attached and in good condition – his biggest fear following the operation had been of pain. Remarkably, he had felt no pain at all.

We had another wait, however. The results of the biopsy were to come. When they arrived, there was no doubt about the diagnosis. It was definitely bowel cancer.

We were more prepared this time. Once again my diary records, 'We have steep hills to climb. It is wonderful not to feel alone.' On my way back from the hospital I stopped at a garden centre and bought a tray of blue Anemone Blanda and planted them in a corner of the garden as a gesture of hope. Now they are spreading. My diary records that I received or made thirty-seven phone calls, did three loads of washing and mended a light fitting. Adrenalin is a wonderful thing, but there is always the need to come down to earth again.

David came home a week after surgery and a short while before Easter. Two days later we were walking to the beach together. He was in great spirits and wanted to get out his paints. A neighbour had mown the lawn in his absence. I had kept a speaking engagement which went well and it was wonderful to come home to him. These were precious days. David often said that he hoped that I would not give up my speaking. We both felt settled and held in a peace beyond our understanding. We went to church together to give thanks. It was an encouragement and a joy to those who had been praying for his recovery, to see him looking so much himself so soon after surgery.

With the operation behind us we were moving on. The question remained of where we were going next. The main thing was that David was alive. What we had to do now – both patient and carer – was to make the most of every day and learn to live with cancer.

As the shock of the diagnosis faded, we became aware of the shock absorbers: people and things that helped to steady us over the months and years that followed. Faithful friends and the closeness of family; the garden and walks by the estuary; the bird life, music and hobbies such as cricket, singing and painting; keeping a diary, private prayer and corporate worship; homemade food – all these presented opportunities to foster the positive side of the life we still had together. There was still so much to enjoy.

One of the most treasured and effective shock absorbers is to have a spiritual director or soul friend. David and I had consulted different people over many years. The person I originally consulted was and is a priest. He provided a safe and regular place where I could lay down some of my burdens and know that I was understood and valued and, if necessary, corrected. He helped me to look for God in some challenging situations, and enabled me to grow in my faith without pushing or coercing me. We laughed a lot. My will was held intact and I felt safe. This involved mutual trust and respect. Eventually this soul friend moved further south and, as we were staying in the north-west, the distance became too great to be practical. We agreed to conclude our sessions but remained friends. I owe him more than I can say.

Around the time in David's journey with cancer, when we knew that the end was in sight, I decided to look for another person to fill this role. After some time, I found one. I chose to consult a priest slightly removed from my own church who knew and respected David. He agreed to see me on a regular basis. I asked him to help me to let David go. It was essential to my spiritual health and general well-being to be able to give account and to unburden systematically to someone who could listen and observe from a more detached position, and who could discern whether or not I was being authentic or whether I was putting on an act. There is a place for putting on a brave face in public, but not at the expense of facing reality in the private place. I fancy that having this safe place also saved me from the neurosis of spraying my concerns around and becoming exhausted with repeating myself, or boring people, or confused by varied advice. Here for an hour each month I could be myself in a structured environment and take stock without being judged.

As David and I were facing an imminent parting, which had been my greatest fear, I asked this priest to help me look for God in every situation however tough. The hour I spent with him each week became a place where I could confess things I was ashamed of, and where I could weep without fear of being overwhelmed with a suffocating sympathy or religiosity, or told to pull myself together. Here I could laugh at myself and we could laugh together. These sessions continue. It has become a place of accountability on earth without judgement; a place of encouragement and insight without sentimentality; a place where I feel respected as a human being and never patronised. It is a place full of wisdom and common sense, where I can rebalance myself after particular traumas. I am helped to do my own growing up. Overall it is a safe place, a place in which God's pure love and mercy are being channelled. It is a hallowed friendship that has been a lynchpin in helping me to take each new step in the adventure of life.

The garden in the spring of 2001 was a total comfort and joy. It was one of the most effective shock absorbers of all. We had put in the work together and now it was responding. A conversation with this little corner of creation was in progress, and that conversation has continued to this day. There we both found a different kind of companionship. Fresh air, birdsong and busy bees, the excitement of seeing and eating fruit and vegetables that we had grown, and the heady and healing scents from lavender, roses, lilies, myrtle and the damp aromatic foliage of cistus and herbs after rain in summer. There was colour to stir the emotions. Reds, pinks, yellows, whites and blues set in a backdrop of relaxing greens made up the palette. There was texture and shape with the sculptural sword-like leaves of phormium and the soft misty blooms of cotinus or smoke bush. Apple blossom promised fruit in autumn. Gifts from friends were everywhere reminding us that we were not alone. The garden beckoned us to dig, weed and wander, but also to sit and ponder with a drink or a meal and enjoy it together and with friends. I thank my mother for her enthusiasm for gardening during the testing times of the Second World War and her asthma-filled days. She showed me, as a small child, the benefits that gardening could bring not only to herself and her family, but to all who entered it, in good times and in bad. David's mother, too, loved her garden. She had been widowed young and was a wonderful example of what love of gardening can do to heal the hurts that life can bring and to fill the vacuum of loss.

Each day I would write my journal quite fully on A4 paper, starting with the immediate and being as descriptive and truthful as possible, and occasionally including my feelings. This proved to be invaluable when the going got tough. The journal became a patient un-judging friend who was there day or night, and who absorbed all that I offered without having hysterics or giving advice. Often after writing, sometimes in the middle of the night, problems would unravel themselves and the way through would open up. It was a kind of prayer to an ever present, ever listening, ever loving God.

By now we had a list of seventeen A4 pages with the names of people who had sent good wishes, including offers of help. This gave us so much strength. We were happily overwhelmed by the kindness of people. One of the offers was from a local clergyman and his wife. They said if there was anything they could do, like offering a meal, I was to ask.

One day I took up their offer, and invited myself to lunch. Much later on, friends in our road invited me to have a delicious breakfast in their kitchen with them from time to time when David was in hospital. These were mini-respites and were delightful ways of starting the day before the chores and the visiting took hold.

Although my mother had settled into her nursing home she needed me to visit regularly. The phone was busy. Quite soon I realised that if our home was to be a peaceful place where my patient could relax, and the carer could remain in one piece, I had to make friends with the answerphone. Telephone calls should not be allowed to become a series of interruptions; instead, I could choose to regard the answerphone as a vehicle for kindness to be received graciously, and I needed to make this happen.

I quickly realised that most people simply wanted to have news of David's progress, and not necessarily a long conversation with me. So I composed a message. It was to be an upbeat, short but truthful bulletin for callers, which thanked them for calling, and gave a brief outline of how the patient was faring. At the same time I asked callers to leave their name and number so that I could ring back later. I realised that there might be calls from other people too, so David was referred to as 'the patient', for purposes of preserving some privacy. In the evening I listened to each message, listing every call so that David could share in the torrent of goodwill when I visited him in hospital. This was a wonderful experience to look forward to at the end of the day.

Consequently I was not stressed by the phone, and did not turn into a long-playing record or an exhausted butterfly repeating information throughout the day. It also gave priority to conversations with those who were visiting us. Most people understood and appreciated the idea. The phone and the answerphone became a conduit of blessings instead of a series of interruptions. It was also good for me as I had to encapsulate the news briefly and succinctly, renewing the automated message twice a day to be up to date. It helped me to focus on the positive, whatever was happening.

It was a blow, though not totally unexpected, to be told that David was to have six months of chemotherapy treatment. This would ground us, reducing our boundaries. It would mean regular trips to the hospital each fortnight where David would be attached to a drip. I went with him and came to appreciate the space to sit down and relax while waiting. I would take mending, letters and cards to write or a book to read. We were in good company and got to know some of the other patients. Although the department was in a certain amount of disruption due to redevelopment, the nurses kept their heads and we felt in safe hands. Only once did we discover that the drug was dripping onto the floor because a wire had come loose.

Chapter 9

Twists and Turns

Brother, sister let me serve you
Let me be as Christ to you:
Pray that I may have the grace
To let you be my servant too.[14]

Meanwhile I was struggling with another challenge. I had accepted an invitation the previous year to be the key speaker at a residential conference for the clergy spouses of Chester Diocese. It was due to start in a fortnight. There were five addresses to be delivered and my time for preparation had been reduced. The start of the conference was uncomfortably close to David's return home from hospital. He was keen for me to keep the engagement but I could not leave him alone. Elisabeth Forster who was organising the conference was most understanding and said that I could leave the decision until a fortnight before the conference was due to begin.

I sounded out my sister Hazel in Ireland, who was a nurse. To our delight, she readily agreed to come to be with David while I was away. So I agreed to keep the engagement. I set about picking up my preparation, but it was difficult to make time to withdraw and to concentrate. Visitors came and went. My mother needed a visit and I was tired and anxious.

The Sunday afternoon before the conference I was panicking and in tears of exhaustion and desperation. I was upstairs struggling with my preparation and time was passing. David was downstairs watching *Songs of Praise*. We usually watched together, and we would often sing along with the hymns. I came down to join him. My throat could only produce strangled sounds and I was fighting with tears. I was in a quandary. Should I worry him with my problem? I knew that he was keen to support me and he was in good form. So somehow it seemed natural to share my anxiety with him once the programme was over. My patient quickly reassured me, believing that I could and would manage the conference, and suggested a session in the morning to look at my work when I was fresher.

This did the trick. David had cared for the carer. My patient had gifts. With a new kind of confidence I set off with only three talks out of five prepared but ready to risk, and with an opportunity to let go; to let go to God, to my hearers and to the situation. I resolved to give my best, however incomplete. The subject was the Friendship of Christ. This included friendship with God, with one another and with oneself.

I was then moved to write a long prayer/poem in the form of a conversation with God. It helped to focus my thoughts on what was important. This is an extract.

> Dear Lord,
> I'm all of a twitter this morning
> My head is in a flat spin
> The women are coming tomorrow
> For some time-out together, but no gin.

My Friend's reply started:

> Sit still, my dear daughter, beside me,
> And see how the matter will pass.
> I am here in the mess and the muddle
> Beside you, from first until last.[15]

Prayer can be a way of 'doing' friendship.

The weekend before I left for the conference there was a knock on the door. There stood a friend with a casserole in his hands. 'This is leek and potato soup. I made it myself. I hope it helps.' An angel on the doorstep had come to our rescue at the perfect moment. I flung my arms round his neck, burst into tears of gratitude and said, 'You angel!' From then on I began my list of angels: people who offered help of all kinds, with their phone numbers. Offers to help included shopping, sitting, driving, meals, 'anything day or night'. It is still on my kitchen cupboard years later as a reminder of the world of kindness and good stories that is in full swing, just under the surface of the rather different world as it is presented so often in the media.

The conference came and went. It was a fulfilling time with a lot of fun. Several people suggested that all the material for a book was there and that I should write it. I accepted that with gratitude and filed the material away.

David meanwhile was continuing to write his autobiography[16] for three hours a day. This kept him focused. My priority was to support him in this, reading and editing his work at his invitation, as it emerged, and as he had done for me years ago.

Spring 2002 turned into summer. David's chemo was producing negligible side effects, apart from tiredness which had lifted by the following afternoon when he mowed the lawn. After each treatment which was tedious, we decided to do something positive by way of a small treat. Sometimes this meant buying an ice cream or having tea out at a nearby garden centre, or picking fresh raspberries at a Pick Your Own field nearby and eating them with cream when we got home.

The cricket season was in full swing so we drove south to stay with David's sister Mary for a few days and to watch his old team Sussex play at the County Ground in Hove. The pollen count was high and I was struggling as usual with my annual trial of hay fever.

The surgeon had told us that David could have five more years. Life was good and we treasured it. It was enhanced by the faithful support of so many friends and family. We felt in good company, and I began to be aware of the strength to be gained by belonging to the community of saints not just in heaven, but on earth. My answerphone strategy was working beautifully.

There followed some good months. The summer was humming. David completed his autobiography and I was very busy organising his book tour which would involve fifteen venues across the country and a good deal of travelling. Like so many fellow cancer sufferers, he was able to carry on fairly normally despite the chemo. This also had to be organised in other venues as we travelled. We were able to holiday in West Wales, where we prepared for the tour by relaxing and painting in a favourite seaside town for a couple of weeks, before getting on the road.

After three years in the writing, David's book *Steps Along Hope Street* was launched in Liverpool Cathedral on 4 October 2002. There was a good deal of interest.

Five days before we were due to set off for the tour, the roller coaster took a dive. The results of David's latest scan showed lesions on his liver. I went cold when I heard this. To me, liver cancer spelt the end. But ignorance is not always bliss. The consultant surgeon was upbeat and told us that the cancer was operable. He also informed us that the liver regenerates itself within a year, which neither of us knew! A date was set for the operation after the tour was completed.

With the schedule in place, we set off carrying this news privately, for a heart-warming two months of signing, speaking, and sleeping in many different beds. I did most of the driving and co-ordinating and David's resilience never ceased to amaze me.

In many ways it was fortuitous for both of us that there was such a demanding task to complete while living with this news. It gave us something else on which to focus our minds. The roller coaster sped on with more thrills and spills. A book event was due to take place one evening in Eastbourne. We were staying with friends in nearby Brighton. Suddenly David became ill with a very high temperature and no energy. We paid an emergency visit to a nearby hospital and explained the predicament. His blood count had dropped drastically. To our astonishment we were told that there was a chance that after some tests he could be treated in time to keep the engagement in Eastbourne inside a couple of hours. We held our breath and waited.

I lived on the mobile, keeping our host in Eastbourne informed of progress while we waited for David to be seen, tests done and treatment administered. The event organiser had to entertain the waiting audience for the best part of an hour until David was released from hospital. I drove like a maniac to deliver him to the patient crowd. He delivered his short talk and signed books till past 10.30 p.m. with a temperature of over 100. By the following morning he had recovered, and we went on to another event. During the whole tour he signed over a thousand books.

The tour over, we returned home. We both took part in singing the *Messiah* with the St Peter's Singers. It was a wonderful way to face a major operation – singing Hallelujah! On 1 December 2002 a quarter of David's liver was removed. Six days later he was home again and had made an excellent recovery. My sister Evelyn joined us for a quiet and peaceful Christmas together. My mother, ninety-two by now, had become very frail and was barely able to recognise us. Her roller coaster was slowing down.

But ours was taking off again.

Chapter 10

Something to Swear About

'Damn! Damn! Damn! Damn!'[17]

The year 2003 saw some nosedives and some sharp turns in the journey. After a long innings, my mother died aged ninety-two. Family members came up for her funeral on the Wirral and later we all gathered for a Thanksgiving Service in her home church in Dorset. David gave the address at both. His health was holding up remarkably well.

The roller coaster then lurched into another dive. We went into Liverpool for a check-up with the consultant following the liver operation and the results of a recent scan. His bowel and liver were clear, but cancer had spread to his lungs. Small pea-sized spots were showing. More chemo was prescribed, this time through an intravenous catheter, a Hickman Line. We left the consultation in a blur. It was a cold and wet May evening. We walked into the driving rain to find the car. The question was what to do next. Should we go home and lick our wounds of disappointment and try to manage the news alone, or was there perhaps another option? I had realised that our local Light Operatic Society in West Kirby, which had an excellent reputation, was performing *My Fair Lady* at the Empire Theatre in Liverpool. Suddenly this seemed like a good idea. 'Let's go!' I said, and David quickly agreed. This sent a shaft of light through the gloom. There was just enough time to dash into the city, park the car and buy tickets. We stood in line at the Box Office. It was already 7.30 p.m. Feeling quite excited by now, hoping we were not too late, we paid and took our seats. It was a brilliant production and we were able to enter into the performance and let the bad news simmer for a little while longer.

When Professor Higgins declared with passion, 'Damn! Damn! Damn! Damn!' in very different circumstances, we felt like joining in. It was a gift, and we let out some of the pent-up emotion with wry knowing glances.

So often we are presented with a fork in the road in life's journey. One way is pointing towards a negative route and the other towards a more positive option. On this occasion we were enabled to choose the positive. The next day we drove to our favourite place in Wales for a pre-booked self-catering holiday, singing, 'Damn! Damn! Damn! Damn!' as we went. There is a time to swear, and a time to refrain from swearing. Expressing our indignation like that was a kind of prayer. It was like saying, 'O God No! Whatever next – just as things were going so well?'

On this occasion 'Damn' drew the sting of potential bitterness. We had taken our books and paints, and we thanked God for the timing of this break. We spoke a little, in short bursts, about facing the end-times. But mostly we enjoyed the fresh air and the break, and the freedom from hospital visits.

Jamie

Less than a month after our return from Wales there was a phone call. David's only nephew, Jamie aged forty-six, had been diag-nosed with a grade 4 brain tumour. He had been given a fortnight to live – fourteen days in which to tell his young family, bid farewell to his friends and leave his business affairs in order. His mother Mary, David's sister, had been told immediately – and had to keep the dreadful news to herself.

Jamie's wife Jo had died from cervical cancer a few years previ-ously.[18] His own imminent death would mean that their three children, between the ages of ten and sixteen, would be left orphaned. We were in shock. David wept. This was tragedy. Where was God in all this? Part of the answer came later.

We were invited for lunch in the family's Oxfordshire garden on a glorious summer day. The meal had been prepared by Jamie's sister-in-law Tessa, who had lost her sister Jo five years ago. She had some time ago agreed, along with her husband Guy, to become guardians to the family. None of them dreamed that it would ever be necessary but they proved to be the perfect choice.

Tessa had been on holiday abroad with her mother when she heard the news of Jamie and came straight back. She and Guy had then moved swiftly into the family home to be with the children.

Jamie was in good form during the lunch. His son Alexander was celebrating his tenth birthday with a party that day. David was asked to say grace. After a moment's hesitation he suggested that Jamie, being the host, should say grace himself. Jamie was not used to this, but immediately took up the invitation. Instead of a short formal, 'For what we are about to receive' kind of grace, Jamie took a deep breath and there followed a natural outpouring of thankfulness to God for his life, his family and his friends, with tears running down his cheeks. This was a heartfelt prayer from a young man who knew he had only days to live, and who was preparing to break the news to his children the following day when they would all be together.

That evening, as the village church bell tolled for evening prayer, Jamie said he would like to go to church. He then decided he couldn't cope. Tessa's husband Guy was a priest and gave him communion sitting in the garden – just the two of them under a huge spreading beech tree. The knowledge of those special moments brought great comfort to Tessa and Guy as they took up their new role of caring for Jamie's family.

Twelve hours later Jamie was in a coma. While on the way for tests the following morning, he suffered a massive seizure. They stopped at the nearest hospital where he went into a coma, and was transferred to a London hospital. As soon as David heard that Jamie was so near the end, he obtained permission from his oncologist to defer his next chemo treatment to the end of the week. He took the train to London to be with his nephew. The following day Jamie died peacefully with his Uncle David by his side.

David's sister Mary made a positive decision not to go to her son's bedside at the end. She knew her limits and did not want her good memories of her son to be overlaid with other images. Someone who knows their limits and goes on to make an appropriate decision has a lot to teach us about staying positive, and about survival. This decision had an important consequence. As a result of it, David felt released to step in and be present, not only as an uncle to Jamie and a brother to Mary, but also as a priest. People undergoing chemo have gifts to offer.

David was asked to compile the funeral service and to preach at both the funeral and the Thanksgiving Service later on, as he had done for Jo previously. This meant a good deal of preparation, thought and travelling. He had to draw deeply on his professional resources in order to manage the inevitable emotion as well as the work involved. By now he was in the middle of a course of chemotherapy and had to pace himself carefully to counter the exhaustion. He struck just the right notes in both services and we were all proud of him.

Tessa and Guy eventually left their home in Bradford and moved two hundred miles to be with Jamie and Jo's children. Guy gave up his job as an archdeacon and they moved in permanently. Never was there a more poignant example of self-giving love in action. Was this a reflection of God's nature in practice? I think it was. There is no greater love.

The children played their part by accepting the tragic news with awesome courage, as did David's sister Mary, for whom the loss of her only son was a major tragedy. Jamie's sister Sarah, who had a fine singing voice, despite her great loss, had the courage to sing at his funeral. Everyone worked hard to adjust to the devastating news, and to play their part in supporting the children. We in the family felt privileged to witness such love in action. They have since thrived in every way.

Chapter 11

Roller Coaster

If I ascend to heaven, thou art there!
If I make my bed in Sheol, thou art there!
If I take the wings of the morning and dwell in the
uttermost parts of the sea, even there thy hand shall lead me,
and thy right hand will hold me.[19]

David resumed his treatment. During the months following Jamie's death, our roller coaster climbed to a high point. Sussex County Cricket Club, which David had captained, won the County Championship for the first time in their 164-year history. This was a timely boost in our household. In 2001 David had been appointed President. To top it all came the announcement that Liverpool had been selected to become the European Capital of Culture in 2008. We felt on top of the world.

We found ourselves giving thanks for so many little things. Our fig tree had produced luscious fruit at last and the sunsets over the estuary were dramatic. Oranges and flaming reds swept the sky and were reflected in the watery sandbanks below. One day we sat by our small pond and, within half an hour, witnessed the emergence of a dragonfly from its chrysalis on a leaf. Even dragonflies have to struggle to find freedom.

With a little shake, its gossamer wings stretched out, sparkling like silk in the sunlight. It was free to fly. But first it remained quite still, as though revelling in the new feeling of freedom and warmth. Then it flew away. It was good to be alive.

It became important to savour these times and let them sink into our total beings. Such times kept our senses alive to beauty and wonder, and enabled us to look for God in the little things on our doorstep. They helped to generate a habit of marvelling, and opened our eyes and ears to all that creation had to offer. Our minds were refreshed and freed from focusing on the next medication, dressing or hospital visit. These precious times could be a diversion from pain for David and from exhaustion for me. It was as though we were banking resources for when the going became tougher. So it proved.

David's continuing walks by the Dee Estuary each morning before breakfast paid dividends with regard to his fitness, together with a modest exercise routine which we undertook together most days. His ability to bounce back after each operation astonished the medics who said he had the muscle tone of a 21-year-old. He was disciplined, and observed his routine with no fuss. He read Morning Prayer and his Bible each day. His siesta in the afternoon had stood him in good stead over many years. In between there was no holding him. He enjoyed his food, his appetite was good and I loved to cook for him. He lived life with relish and energy, but with a large dose of common sense thrown in.

The cards and phone calls kept coming, wishing David well and assuring us of the prayer and love of so many. We were not allowed to feel alone. This was, indeed, the friendship of Christ in action.

The cancer spots on his lungs progressed, so David was fitted with a syringe driver which was a small pump in a box-like contraption that constantly administered strong drugs. This hung round his neck and tucked inside his shirt and was attached to a line into his chest.

In September 2003 there were two further setbacks, the major one being the shattering news that David's friend and colleague Jim Thompson had died. Jim had recently retired as Bishop of Bath and Wells and had suffered a stroke while on holiday with Sally his wife, and died. We travelled to the Thanksgiving Service in Wells Cathedral in which David took part. By this time, he had two fistula drainage bags attached to his abdomen, and an abscess had erupted.

Nevertheless he was as determined as ever to live fully within this new set of boundaries. In October 2003 the intravenous catheter was eventually removed, and David amazed us all by returning to take his seat in the House of Lords in December. He received a great welcome.

There was some respite over Christmas and until the spring of 2004. David was in great form, but then things began to decline more rapidly. The spots on the lungs had progressed even further and a new tumour had appeared in the bowel. We learnt that it was 'the size of a cricket ball'. There were frightening attacks of pain during the night and vomiting. Twice I rang the doctor on night duty. Then I contacted NHS Direct. An ambulance arrived, and David was driven away to hospital as an emergency. More surgery followed for another bowel resection in order to remove the 'cricket ball'. The surgeon could not have been more helpful.

Two infections followed which weakened him noticeably and he was eventually sent home. Then, suddenly, our next-door neighbour died after a short illness, to the shock of all in our road who knew him. It was a see-saw of a summer, and we dipped into our reserves.

There had come a point during the summer of 2004 when at last it seemed the right moment to ask the prognosis question. David never suggested asking it until then, and I had felt that it was right to wait until he was ready.

Jenny was with us when the consultant surgeon called in to see us. The questions were put to her. 'How long have I got?' 'How long have we got with him?' She told us frankly, and with great sensitivity, that David would probably be with us for Christmas 2004 in five months time, and if we were lucky he would have a month or two more after that.

This completely changed the landscape. After the consultant left there were tears and the three of us clung to each other. Now we knew. Instead of concentrating on living with cancer, we now had to prepare to let each other go. We had to meet the hitherto unwelcome visitor, death, without fear and with as much readiness as we could muster. This would be a different journey for each of us. Above all, there had to be dignity, quality of life, comfort and sensitive loving for David. His body bore the wounds of the many physical trials of the past months, and he had fallen three times. He was becoming less mobile. Soon he would have to leave our bed for the last time and come downstairs to our sun-room where he would occupy a hospital bed. This would make the nursing easier.

After the consultant's visit, we decided to have a break and then to talk together that evening to share our thoughts and feelings.

This was a crucial conversation and helped us to move on to the next stage of accepting the inevitable. David's first thought was to ask me what I would do after he had gone. I tried to tell him. Later I made a list of what I would miss about him, and also of my interests and of the people closest to me. He seemed reassured. Talking helps when facing fears. It is tempting to put this off, till for some it is too late. Also, I found writing things down helped to crystallise thoughts and to bring them from the realm of the imagination into reality.

By this time the blanket chest on the landing was like a super-market shelf, with boxes of dressings, rubber gloves and fistula drainage bags piled high. Downstairs in the kitchen I had made an elaborate chart showing which drugs to administer and when. David had two bags attached to his abdomen which needed regu-lar attention, day and night, and the syringe driver.

I learnt to empty and change the fistula bags for him as he was content for me to do this. The procedure involved patience from both patient and carer and was not something to be done in a hurry. Each area had to be cleaned, disinfected and dried and the bags emptied of discharged material, or changed. It meant paying special attention to the skin which had become so sensitive from repeated peeling of the plastic attached to the abdomen. The used bags then had to be emptied into a plastic jug or disposed of into another bag designated for the purpose. We bought some jogging trousers with drawstrings to minimise any chafing of the area. The district nurse came in regularly in the daytime and was a real support and encouragement to us both.

Gradually David was losing his strength and it was clear that another stage had been reached. He was the most patient of patients and his suffering grace was most inspiring to me and helped to keep my motivation high during some testing times.

Once in the middle of the night I emptied and changed his bags as usual and placed the plastic jug with its contents on the bed-room floor while helping him back to bed after a time on the commode. Then I knocked the jug over. It was 3 a.m. and the carpet was cream.

Fortunately David went back to sleep quickly and did not witness the silent disaster. Nor was he disturbed by the conse-quent clearing up, down on my hands and knees, using two whole rolls of kitchen paper and a brush, giving the carpet a good scrub. Remarkably there is no sign of that incident on the carpet today. But it is etched in my memory. David had an expression for a new disaster: 'What a palaver!' It kept us smiling. I whispered it under my breath.

Visitors brought variety and cheer. Most people were sensitive and left before tiring the patient. Just occasionally, one or two out of nervousness talked too much, which became awkward. I eventually greeted visitors at the door, telling them that after ten minutes we might turf them out! They always took the hint with good humour.

One of the happiest visits was from four of David's veteran cricket colleagues from the Sussex County Cricket Club. Rupert Webb, who initiated the visit, was accompanied by Alan Oakman, Jimmy Parks and Kenny Suttle. Although clearly thinner and weaker by now, David rose to the occasion and joined in the reminiscing and the cricket stories, loving every minute of the encounter. Cricket became one of the best pain relievers! These four men had gone to considerable trouble in travelling to come to see their friend. They had made an effort to be there. This kind of friendship brings joy and laughter in the meeting, and also brings a healing of the spirit to an ailing body. It brings peace. A few weeks later, Kenny Suttle died.

David and I were thankful for our spiritual directors who provided each of us with a safe place in which to explore our attitudes to death and dying and to letting a loved one go. There was more life to be lived yet. For some of us, even the end times can be golden, provided we treasure every moment as if it was the last. Joy can arise out of grief.

Each year in Liverpool Cathedral there is a service for those who have lost loved ones to cancer. It is an opportunity for all who wish to come together, religious believers or not, to remember those who have died and to hear their names read out. In 2004 David was to give the address.

The day before the service he was in acute pain and we were gravely concerned that he might have to cancel. But from somewhere he found the will and the energy, and decided to go ahead.

We had acquired a wheelchair to transport him to his seat to conserve his energy, and friends nearby made their home available before and after the service for rest and refreshment. The main body of the cathedral was full and we all held our breath as he mounted the steps to the lectern. Though clearly a sick man, he delivered his address standing tall, with a strong voice and many were moved by his words and by his courage.

The original plan had been to leave David in his seat at the end of the service until the procession had moved off, in order to save him walking. I felt that, as he had done so well, and that with his adrenalin up, he might like to do the normal thing and join the procession as a final act of farewell. The civic party began to move. I threw convention to the winds and walked swiftly across the floor to ask him if he would like to process if I walked beside him. He said that he would.

David was robed in his purple cassock but he had lost weight. As he stood up his wide sash, the purple cincture, slipped from around his waist, and fell to the ground. With no time to pick it up and fix it, I whispered in his ear to step out of it, which he did most deftly. We moved forward together, leaving the sash on the floor, and caught up with the procession. David walked down the long aisle that he had first travelled, alone and unattended, twenty-nine years ago, to be enthroned as the bishop. He departed, this time, enveloped in a new fellowship. He was a human being, in solidarity with people who lived with cancer. There was a ripple of gentle affectionate applause and some tears as he passed. Jenny was waiting with the wheelchair and David left the cathedral for the last time. I resolved never to leave his side till he left mine.

Chapter 12

The Preparation and the Pattern

... underneath are the everlasting arms ...[20]

Three days after his final act of ministry in the cathedral, David was admitted to hospital for an ileostomy which left him with an opening in the abdomen. Surgery had been delayed as had been agreed beforehand between his surgeon and ourselves, so that he could see this commitment at the cathedral through. The operation relieved one problem but he gradually became visibly weaker.

Facing your own death is one thing. Facing the death of a loved one is quite another. Both involve a letting go. Issues surrounding death now seemed to be staring me in the face because my awareness had been heightened. I believe that, in the mercy of God, I had been prepared to some extent and in various ways over the years. It is only in retrospect that I can see this and there was still much to learn.

Life had taken on a different complexion now that the prognosis question had been raised and we knew the answer. Our landscape had changed. We changed. The road ahead came into focus. Life had been precious before, but now every minute counted. Senses were heightened. Colours became more vivid, and flavours more intense. We cherished family members and friends more than ever and we discovered yet again a world of kindness in action. Much of that kindness was to be found in our road, in our church, in the National Health Service and further afield.

Death appeared in the news, in conversations, in books, in people's stories and even in the hymns in church. It seemed to be following me around. This was disconcerting at first, as we had been concentrating on life and the quality of life. I could choose to run away and hide from this taboo subject, avoiding its implications. I could take a half-look at it, like a small child peeping from behind a chair when viewing *Dr Who* on the television. Or I could face it. The choice was mine.

But there was no getting away from it. Losing David had been my greatest fear, so this was a major challenge. We had survived the last three years of living with his cancer, since the initial diagnosis. We had survived better than we had dared hope. Apart from being grounded for chemo, David had shown great resilience. He had continued to live a full and creative life within the new boundaries, overcoming the setbacks when they appeared. Even the medics commented on this.

I had learnt new skills and rearranged priorities. This new life contained real joy amid the sorrow. Instead of a sense of impending doom, we were enabled to see that each change of the fistula bag, or visit to the commode, was an opportunity for love to transform the situation, by the way this was managed.

I remembered watching a care assistant in my mother's nursing home feeding her with such unhurried gentleness, with a teaspoon. I had been transfixed. It was a holy moment. I felt that this was the friendship of Christ in action. I wanted to be like that with my beloved patient.

Now it was time to acknowledge that David was not superhuman. Within a few months his physical decline would accelerate. His spirit though was strong and it was shining through. But we now needed to begin to lay down our metaphorical arms and give in graciously to the inevitable; to give in, in the most positive way, and to accept that death was on its way.

Quality of life and maintaining David's dignity was paramount. I began to see body, mind and spirit as distinct from one another, though connected. In squaring up to the inevitability of David's death, I became less afraid. A 'half-look' would have been much more frightening, leaving a chink through which imagination could play havoc.

The need to face up to realities had come home to me some years before, during a break in Scotland when we stayed in a small croft in Argyll. Our water supply came from the hill behind us. Rainwater passed down the hillside and into an old bath, and on through a pipe into a large metal tank, and then into our taps.

One day the water appeared to dry up although outside it was pouring with rain. We went to investigate. In the bath there appeared to be something floating, blocking the pipe between the bath and the tank. At first glance I thought I saw a severed human hand with fingers waving in the water. I turned away in distress and passed the buck to David, asking him to deal with it. He was not as upset as I, and he had a proper look. It was not a human hand after all. It was a little drowned frog. David removed the frog and the water gushed out into the empty tank.

That experience taught me to realise that it pays to look what frightens us full in the face. I am reminded of the wise words of a friend: 'Block the imagination till the facts come through.' Imagination and knee-jerk reactions can play tricks on us. We see things that are not there. However, once confronted with the facts we can decide what to do without necessarily running away. I recall the words of the Scottish Jesuit Gerry Hughes some years ago: 'The facts are kind.' The frog incident served as a corrective in helping me to face reality. It was a key piece in the jigsaw of preparing to face my greatest fear.

It was time to prepare ourselves for letting David go. He would have his own battle to fight. My job as carer would become more demanding and I was ready for that. Already there had been some mini-bereavements.

When David suffered an infection which left him unable to talk intelligibly, I grieved deep down, thinking that it was the end of our ability to have a normal conversation. Mercifully, the infection cleared and his ability to talk clearly returned. After the second bout of chemo, he lost his hair and I knew that it would never return. Privately I wept. I loved his hair. His legs began to give way and he fell several times. To witness this strong man weakening with both courage and grace, was heartbreaking. These were times of real loss, and the bereavement process was beginning well before his death.

I became aware of the smaller bereavements as part of the larger picture and was unafraid to show emotion privately. Little by little, this helped towards the final parting. I had to come to terms with the fact that the nature of the journey was now about quality of life and comfort for the patient. It was not, primarily, about my loss. This helped me to focus on conserving my energy in order to provide what was needed when it was needed. At the same time, it was important to attend to my own needs.

I was able to deposit my tears and anxiety discreetly and in various ways. So grief was expressed and dissipated rather than being allowed to build up. This, in turn, made way for increased energy with which to concentrate on caring. It was important for me to seek ways of retrieving my balance promptly after the very stressful times. This is where my daily journal became a faithful and discreet friend.

My daughter has great gifts of common sense and empathy and we grieved together. There was also a handful of trusted friends that I could ring when I needed a listening ear. Sometimes a spell in the garden did the trick, or a walk by the river. Letting go little by little was good preparation for the final moment of parting.

Each loss involved the need to stay with the pain and then move on. David's bald head now issued a challenge to me. Unlike me, he appeared to accept it without a problem. Either I could look at it and mourn the loss of his hair till I indulged in self-pity, or I could shed a few tears privately and then let go and make something positive out of it. As his hair fell out in handfuls I combed it gently, and removed all traces of it from his pillows and pyjamas with a small gadget. In my family, when we were children at bedtime my mother had brushed our hair one hundred times with a Mason Pearson hairbrush. We loved this time together when Mum slowed down and gave us her whole attention, often in front of the fire. I had hoped that David would enjoy the attention, in the same way, though without the hundred brushstrokes, and he did. In this way I found joy out of the sorrow, and closeness out of potential distance.

Little overwhelmings are healthy and releasing. But staying too long with the pain can affect the health and focus of the carer and therefore the quality of care for the patient. It can be the spring-board to self-pity. I did not want to go there. I never liked it in others. David had never showed self-pity and there was no reason why I should.

All through this journey I had felt it was important to look for David's motivation and move with it. I needed to spot what he wanted and to bolster his will – his will to live. This became almost a game. His lust for life was evident and an inspiration. It would excite me to see him wanting to go for a walk by the estuary while he still could, or down the garden to inspect his beloved compost heap. He wanted to spend time at his desk or read a book; to eat and drink with relish and to enjoy visitors. He loved seeing his grandchildren.

David had always looked forward to singing, and enjoyed our visits to concert hall or theatre. He had relished his trips to London to attend the House of Lords. He had found preparing sermons so much more fulfilling with more time in retirement to think and to read. He never lost his motivation to watch a game of cricket. All this, despite having chemotherapy and radiotherapy and wearing the syringe driver for the drugs. He was coping with the opening on the abdomen because of the ileostomy and with the two fistula bags. His body had become a pincushion.

Death had seemed a long way off in the early years of cancer, but now we knew that the battle was waning. Those few years in retirement brought us very close. At the same time, almost imperceptibly, we were preparing to separate.

I felt myself moving into a new way of looking at life. Death was now part of it and it was natural. I had known all this in my head. Now my heart was involved too. But I was no longer afraid and I was learning to live with a little more mystery. I had been a cancer patient myself in the days before the advanced strides of today in research and treatment. David had cared for me then and I had survived.

Now the tables had turned. Much of what we faced at that time helped us to communicate more easily now. We had confronted the 'What if I died?' questions when I had had cancer eight years into our marriage. Then, with a will, we had been enabled to move back into life. I owed him so much, and now it was my turn to care for him whatever the cost.

I had also been given a taste of what is involved in parting from a loved one through the deaths of my parents and of Jamie. David had lost his father when he was eight years old. But there were new lessons in parting that we had to learn.

Part of my preparation, I believe, was through a painting. One day a local vicar called and asked each of us to paint a picture for his parish exhibition which was to be held in the week running up to Easter called Passion week. He had spotted artistic talent among his congregation, and came to ask if we would join in. We were invited to choose a particular aspect of the story of Christ's Passion from his prepared list. We both agreed to have a go.

I had never painted from imagination before. This was a real challenge. For some strange reason I chose 'The Agony in the Garden' and decided early on not to include the figure of Christ. It would be too difficult. Gradually the picture became too complicated and without a focus. The three crosses of Calvary were in the distance, the disciples were asleep under a tree. Judas was coming over the hill with the soldiers – and so it went on.

They all had to be taken out. I had to begin again and simplify. I had to come back to Christ himself. Having firmly decided that I would not and could not contemplate painting the face of Christ, I found that I was being led to do just that. I decided to paint in tones of dark blue/grey on plain paper. This felt risky.

One evening I asked David to model for me, principally to get an idea of the way the folds of the garment that Christ was wearing would fall. He knelt on the floor dressed in his bishop's rochet – a long white garment – and I asked him to look up and to hold a wine glass high, with both hands, in an act of offering the cup of suffering. I asked him to straighten his elbows to show that the offering was a willing one. I also asked him to look as agonised as possible, which he did well. I made four quick sketches and at last I knew that the picture was beginning to come together.

I would paint Christ kneeling down, offering high up, with fully extended arms, his cup of suffering. I wanted his face to be an 'everyman' face, so that male or female, young or old, could identify with him. The face would be raised to heaven, full of agony, yet full of determination to see this through. Over the cup I painted a hovering dove depicting the blessing of the Holy Spirit. The sky was cloudy, and in the distance was a hill. In the foreground I put a small olive tree with the disciples, asleep in a huddle on the ground. This, I felt, would speak of even his closest friends abandoning him in his hour of need.

But the more I tried to enter into the situation of Jesus' suffering and impending death, the more troubled I became. Surely the God that I believed in did not leave him to suffer like this without any support or source of strength? Something was missing. I went back to St Luke's Gospel to search for clues. It sprang out of the text, like a flash of lightning: a text that I thought I had known for years. 'And the Lord sent an angel to strengthen him.' My anxiety disappeared.

The dove hovering over the cup in blessing became an angel bringing strength to the Saviour of the world in his struggle. In his agony, and in offering up his cup of suffering, he received strength to fulfil his calling. He completed his task. He knows what it feels like to suffer. He understands. He has left us a pattern and a model to follow. There is strength in the struggle for us too. We can look for the angels who are waiting with gifts to strengthen us.

That discovery, through the painting, helped both David and me to offer up our suffering many times. Angels came and ministered to us; very human angels, but angels nonetheless and they strengthened us. God's spirit was with us.

In thinking about death it helped me to have an image of what we are moving on to, however incomplete. If Christianity is about anything, it is about a relationship. We make a start if we believe that we go to a person and a place where we belong, a place in which there is no more sorrow or pain, a place where we will receive a welcome from someone who loves us unconditionally. 'Underneath are the everlasting arms' is a phrase used to describe the truth that God will be there to catch us when we stumble or fall. That God will be a place of safety and security when we die.

This had been vividly and lastingly illustrated for me in an incident involving my father, which was once again to do with friendship. A few years previously, when my father was in his eighties, he attended church one Sunday as usual. He was a modest man and sat at the back of the church unless he was leading the service. His friend sat nearby and noticed that Dad was not looking quite himself. He enquired if he was feeling all right. My father said, a little too robustly, that he was fine.

He went forward for communion as usual and his friend kept an eye on him. When Dad reached the altar rail, he collapsed. His friend was right behind him and caught him in his arms, saving him from injury. He revived and was taken home. The following week he was back in church and his old self.

In such a way we are given glimpses of the friendship of Christ in our friends and in every person who cares for another in genuine love. The story of my father shows how easy it is to cling to our independence, especially late in life, and how easy it is to push our friends away when we fear being a nuisance. My father's friend took no notice of his rebuff, and kept an eye on him. He was there when the independence gave way.

Chapter 13

Letting Go

So the choice for every human being is between death and death –
the death of a letting go that hurts like hell but leads to
resurrection, or the slow extinction as all the energies are spent
on getting and keeping, instead of living and giving.[21]

There is so much that is still mysterious about dying. It helps
though to stop and reflect a while and to talk to one another about
our hopes and fears.

It must be much easier to let go in death if we have some idea
that everything will be all right. If wrongs that we have committed
have been confessed and forgiven, then our consciences will be
clear and any lurking guilt will be assuaged, clearing the way. We
need to feel safe, and that 'the everlasting arms' will be there to
hold us and to keep us from falling for ever. It must also be easier to
let go if we have known what it is to be rescued or held by someone
who loves us, especially when we have been fearful.

But what if, in this life, those arms fail us? What if our friends are
not there when we are falling? What if we fail to be alongside
others through unfaithfulness, laziness or forgetfulness? What if
we have preferred to be totally independent all our lives, but now
find we are unable to cope without help?

If any of those things happens, there is a break in the chain of
belonging. Relationship is harmed. We feel disconnected, alone
and abandoned. We are hurt and we may become angry and
resentful, looking for someone to blame, someone on whom to lay
responsibility for the way we feel.

We may blame ourselves for not making our position clear, for
being too independent. We may strike out in our pain. 'My God
where are you?' 'What do I do now?' 'Where do we go from here?'
'I cannot trust anyone again.' These things happen to human
beings. We fail each other. We let one another down, again and
again. We let ourselves down.

The theologian James Houston tells us: 'Many people today are without friends and without God … we need each other, yet we so readily wound each other.'[22] That is an unfortunate fact which it is better to face.

The need for the bonds of faithful friendship and for security is universal. It is reflected even in the relationship between a man or woman and their dog! Driving through Liverpool's Sefton Park one day I saw a dog dart out in front of a car and be hit by it. The dog was clearly distressed and in great pain. The car stopped immediately and the driver got out to see if he could help. I stopped too and joined him. A small crowd gathered. The injured creature was not able to accept comfort from any of us. We were strangers. One person looked at the dog's collar and went in search of the owner. Soon the owner arrived and knelt beside her beloved dog. Immediately the dog lifted his head, put it in her lap, relaxed and died.

Such incidents can throw light on dying. It is easier to let go with someone who knows us well and loves us dearly.

Our model is Christ himself who lived as a human being, setting aside the joys and security of heaven to be with us and to share our struggles as well as our joys. He revealed the importance of friendship. When the time came to face his own death in unique circumstances, Christ showed us a way of dealing with it. A line in the Thanksgiving Prayer in the Church of England gives a clue: 'The night before he died, he had supper with his friends.' These words have a particular resonance for me as I shall explain in the next chapter.

Christ wanted to spend time with the people closest to him and to leave them important instructions. He was equipping them for his departure, and for their mission when he had left. He broke bread and drank wine using these elements to indicate the kind of death he was to face. His body would be broken and his blood spilt. He also said thank you to his father.

This was a time of intimacy, away from the crowds, and a time of commissioning. Here was an opportunity to say good-bye: a unique God-be-with-you moment. Christ knew that in front of him lay a supremely lonely road which only he could take. His life on earth was complete, and now he knew that his disciples, whom he now called friends, were ready to build on what he had begun.

But they needed to be called in a special way. Their Master was leaving them. As servants they would be lost without him. Christ stepped in with a new way of looking at their relationship with him. This constituted a new vocation for them and a position of trust.

'I call you servants no longer. I call you friends.' With these words he demonstrated something of what he meant when he washed their feet, overturning their image of the Master/Servant relationship as they had known it, and developing it to a more mutual way of living and working. But first they were exhorted to love one another, as he had loved them.

The disciples were moving on from obediently, and perhaps blindly at times, receiving orders or commands from a Lord and Master. They were now learning to be faithful friends and mature human beings, serving and being served; giving and receiving in mutual respect. They were to become friends with God, friends with others and friends with themselves.

Christ had taught them and trained them for this task by example and through conversation. He had demonstrated the qualities of faithful friendship with all kinds of people. He knew that his disciples needed to feel secure after he had gone. So it made sense to reiterate that he would never leave them or forsake them and that he would send them a Comforter to strengthen them.

They had their model. They had had their training. Now they had to grow up and find friends in the nooks and crannies of the world in which there was hurt, disease and need of all kinds. This mission was a tall order, but it came with the resources they needed. They had each other, and they had the Spirit of Christ.

As Jesus hung dying on the cross, his thoughts were for others: for his family and for his fellow sufferers. In pain he shouted at God. He wanted to go home and back to where he belonged. But he left part of himself behind. The Holy Spirit is now our mentor and our friend, as he was for the disciples, helping us to live and to die, through friendship with one another and with creation.

The hospice

One of the places that can teach us to face our fear of dying is the hospice. The founder of the modern hospice movement, Dame

Cicely Saunders, has left us a gift which we must treasure. As David's needs became greater, Jenny and I decided to prepare ourselves for the possible moment when he might be referred. We had both heard about hospices, read about them, but had never visited one. We had in our ignorance come to the conclusion that hospices were places where people only went to die. We made an appointment to visit our local hospice, St John's, on the Wirral, and with some trepidation walked through the doors. David knew nothing about this.

Inside, the hospice was warm and airy. Fresh flowers were in the entrance area and a cheery welcome from a volunteer greeted us at reception. We signed in as visitors.

An hour later, we were ignorant no longer. There was a tranquillity about the place. There were clearly patients who were on their way towards death, but peacefully. Others had come for short stays for pain relief and pain control. The ratio of nurses to patients was high and there were willing volunteers to help with practical tasks and be there when needed. Often these were people who had lost loved ones themselves and had returned out of gratitude for the care received. There was a trained counsellor at hand to sit with patients and also with family members who had questions and worries. There was a day centre where patients could meet each other and have a cup of tea, take part in various artistic and therapeutic activities if they wished. The hospice was a place for all the family. It was a place to learn together how to live with dying. We walked out of the place we had feared in quiet awe, ignorant no longer. We felt prepared. Jenny said quietly, 'It was perfect.'

'Even when we can do absolutely nothing we still have to be prepared to stay,' said the founder. That sums up so much of the reality of hospice care. 'Watch with me' means, above all, 'Just be there', she said. This may sound over-simple. But it is in fact a profound key to a person's peace of mind as we face the greatest letting go of all. We were not designed to be alone.

After a particular episode of pain, the doctor decided that David should be admitted to St John's Hospice for palliative care. He was home after a week, and much more comfortable. There were to be several future visits, each lasting for a week or so.

So with our pattern in place, David and I moved to the next stage. He was now clearly ill and in pain, and Christmas was coming.

On 13 December 2004 David fell again and was admitted to the hospice. He was left-handed and he now found that he could not write with his left hand. He was sent for a brain scan. He was still signing letters that I had prepared, but this time with his right hand.

This development put a cloud over Christmas hopes and plans. Unlike previous visits to the hospice, this time David did not settle. He was unusually tense. It was when he said that he wanted to come home that I knew that he realised he was on the last lap of his journey. He wanted to die at home.

To our great joy, the hospice team worked their palliative magic over eleven days and he came home on Christmas Eve. The family was all together. Christmas Day dawned. Our two grandsons bounded downstairs to find their bulging red stockings on the hearth. David joined us early in the morning as we sipped tea in our dressing gowns, and witnessed the delight of the two small boys in front of the fire. He rested while we attended church. He sat at table with us for Christmas lunch, entering into the festivities wholeheartedly. This was the greatest and most poignant gift for all of us so far. I said to him, 'At this rate you'll be there for my seventieth birthday party!' This was to be three months later. 'I'll be there,' he said firmly. And he was, by a whisker.

I was now battling with exhaustion. I shall not easily forget the feeling of legitimate release and gratitude when a Marie Curie Cancer Care night nurse came to enable me to have some respite. I had to hand over the reins of care to a complete stranger, but knew that I needed to slacken the bow. The idea of this was disturbing at first after caring intensively for so long. But having said goodnight to my dear man, I sank into the spare bed and closed the door at midnight, knowing that he was in safe hands. It was like going on holiday. My niece Jemma came to stay for a few days and was a tower of strength, releasing me to sit with David. She, alone, at that time witnessed some of the raw grief that was privately overcoming me now and again and was a calm and practical support. Jenny and I were in daily contact by phone.

The mini-bereavements were gathering momentum. Having twice resisted the gentle suggestion of the district nurse that David should move downstairs from our bedroom to a hospital bed, we realised that the time had come to give in. This was the last time we would ever share a bed together and it was painful for us both.

The steroids had weakened his muscles so that the stairs were becoming increasingly difficult to manage. One evening it became evident that for the first time he had not the strength to mount them. It was nearly ten o'clock. Realising that I was not strong enough to help him up to bed, I rang Malcolm the curate. He and Tony, a friend from church, were round in minutes and, with their strong arms, helped David up the stairs. It was all done with great humour and gentleness, but inwardly we mourned.

The next day, Jenny and I moved fast and consulted the district nurse. Phone calls were made, and within a day a hospital bed was delivered and placed in our sun-room downstairs in place of our large favourite sofa which had to be put in store to make room for the new arrangement. The room was full of light, faced south-west and was in full view of the garden. One of the spare beds was brought down for me, so that David would not be alone. We made up his bed with new sheets brought by a kind local friend with plenty of pillows. A bedsitter was created with flowers and a new small television.

With enormous courage David insisted on walking down the stairs for the last time, though with some difficulty, with help from two nurses. There was not a dry eye. He walked slowly and deliberately to the bed, with quiet dignity. He climbed in and sank back on the pillows. It was January.

By the end of the day he was watching cricket on Sky TV. For the next few weeks he was glad to receive short visits, but was now bed-bound.

During this time I had been organising my birthday party on 5 March, the day after my seventieth birthday and the day before David's 76th, wondering whether it would happen. Forty invitations had gone out to family and friends. Two weeks before the day, David became weaker. I told him that we could easily cancel the party as people would understand. But he clearly wanted me to go ahead with it. There followed a most extraordinary two weeks when I felt torn between wanting to spend every minute sitting still with him, and yet being very busy with both the caring and the party preparations.

Though David did not talk much about dying, I knew that he believed firmly in life after death and in the resurrection of the body. He believed firmly that he was on his way home, to God. But drugs were being administered and although he was mostly at peace, there were one or two moments of disturbance.

One of the most heart-rending moments came when he suddenly propped himself up in the bed one evening and called out to me across the room: 'Don't leave me. Don't leave me alone. Stay with me. I don't want to be alone.' It was a cry from someone who perhaps had had a glimpse of eternal abandonment. Morphine may also have contributed to the underlying distress.

I went straight over to him, and promised that I would stay with him. He rested back into his pillows. This big strong dependable man that I had lived with for nearly fifty years had reached the lowest point of vulnerability and was allowing it to show. His uncharacteristic cry spoke volumes of the deep-seated need that we have for each other, especially in times of great fearfulness. Christ had spoken to this need when he said to his disciples at supper on the night before he died: 'I will never leave you or forsake you.' What did Christ mean? I think I was to find out later.

The preparations for the party were nearly complete. My sister Evelyn and I bought several metres of cream voile and made a curtain to divide the room, should David need private attention. In the event it was not needed as he was so peaceful. Debbie, who had cooked for our bigger occasions in Liverpool, was producing the food to release me to be with David as much as possible. The house was in order, and beds made up. Overflow hospitality was provided by our kind neighbours. The family arrived. There was a strange subdued excitement at having reached this point in the journey.

It was springtime. Signs of new life in the garden brought hope and anticipation. All hope of David's earthly life continuing much longer had given way to a new kind of hope: that he would die peacefully and be able to reach his goal of being with us at the party.

March 5th dawned. David was still with us.

Chapter 14

The Party and the Parting

On the night before he died he came to supper with his friends and taking bread he gave thanks ...[23]

The day of 5 March 2005 will remain in my memory as a day when joy and sorrow mingled into a creative force. It was the day between our birthdays. He had celebrated his seventy-fifth birthday with a party the previous year and had been keen for me to go ahead with my seventieth. I had been energised by his clear wish to give me joy. We had hoped that those who came would not be embarrassed or fearful, but would somehow be given the gift that David was offering; the gift of being able to say goodbye in a party atmosphere. Our two young grandsons played cricket and football on the lawn outside his window. They were aware of what was happening and were able also to be carefree. It made all the difference to have them with us at such a time.

As I sat at his bedside on the morning of the party, I recalled three phrases that David had uttered frequently in the previous few weeks. He had repeated them as though they were at the forefront of his mind. They were in effect his final words: 'Thank you', 'I love you' and 'Yes!'

Every small act of caring brought a 'Thank you'. 'Yes' demonstrated the positive spirit he showed throughout his cancer journey – it could have been so different.

His spoken declaration of love for me when so weak will remain with me for ever. He could have taken it for granted that I knew that he loved me without mustering the energy to voice it. This expression of his love mirrored the unconditional and eternal love of the suffering Christ for all who accept him. It also provides a basic pattern of worship and has remained as an icon to my faith ever since.

On the morning of the party the house was full of family. Breakfast was cleared. David was ready and resting peacefully. Debbie arrived with her assistant, bringing the food freshly cooked and in dishes ready to serve.

There was an air of excitement and quiet wondering as we approached lunchtime and the arrival of the first guest. I had prepared and printed out a note of explanation for this unusual party which would be handed to each person as they arrived. This would save me repeating myself to each one and they were invited to read it straightaway.

Thank you for coming today.

Having this party is quite barmy on one level.

On another it is utterly appropriate.

What is important is that David wanted me to go ahead with it. So did Jenny.

The doctor and nurses have supported the idea all along.

This occasion has been an important target in David's long journey and we are thrilled that he has been enabled to reach it.

David's phrase 'Let's do it' is one among many that has inspired and strengthened me. So together we've done it! Thank God with us.

Thank you for being with me to celebrate becoming really elderly with style.

Let's celebrate God's gift of life however flickering it sometimes is.

We want to thank you for all your imaginative, unstinting, loving support during this four-year sojourn. You have helped us stay afloat in the most extraordinary way during the last few months: together we have made the most beautiful patchwork out of love and friendship.

Close to journey's end, David is still with us and in the heart of the party. He is in bed, sleeping mostly, in the sun-room. Perhaps you would like to see him, if so, please do come in and sit with him for a minute or two. Otherwise, please be assured that he knows you are here.

We appreciate the varied emotions you may have, but hope you will enjoy yourself, perhaps in a new and surprising way.

All along we have viewed each day as a new adventure.

Each day has had its palavers.

Thank you for being part of this one!

David, Grace and Jenny

We had decided to have three parties in one. It was 'a bit of a palaver' – to use David's phrase which had so often lightened the traumatic moments of the previous four years.

There was a Noisy Party in the kitchen/dining room where there was food and drink, and also a friend playing some favourite music on the piano. There was a Quiet Party across the hall in the sitting room which adjoined the sun-room in which David lay. Here, family, friends and neighbours could come and go, and talk quietly with food on their knees. In the sun-room itself there was a Very Quiet Party where people just sat, or read the newspaper, or chatted in low voices.

One after another came to spend a few moments of farewell, and in private and prayerful communication at David's bedside. I sat nearby most of the time. Just occasionally he was able to identify someone and whisper their name. He clearly knew what was happening though his strength was ebbing away.

The small boys came in as it was getting cool outside and the light was failing. They had been well prepared and included all along, and they brought the gift of innocence to us all. They were not afraid and asked questions when they arose.

It is difficult to describe the atmosphere as emotions were high yet restrained. It was prayerful and natural and without fear.

There was an air of watchful waiting in the house, mixed with laughter and joy. Because we were together, nothing was hidden and no one was excluded. Joy and sorrow combined. Love and loss travelled side by side. We were journeying together and still able to celebrate. Dying and living seemed to belong in the same space.

Once again I was reminded of Christ, our model. 'The night before he died he had supper with his friends.' This line in the eucharistic prayer never fails to move me now. It speaks to me of the party we had – our last supper – and the value of being together with loved ones before death. It speaks, too, of the importance of hospitality: of eating, drinking and talking together, and of remembering.

By early evening, just the family and one or two friends remained. Jenny and I, my sisters and two friends sat nearby, occasionally singing quietly. Someone suggested saying the Lord's Prayer. Chopin Nocturnes were on the CD player.

David's breathing changed and became laboured. In my ignorance, I became anxious that he might suffocate as his lungs were filling up. To prevent further anxiety I phoned the surgery in case there was someone available to enlighten me. Astonishingly, our GP was just leaving and picked up the phone himself. He reassured me that what was happening was natural and that David would not suffocate. Very soon a nurse arrived and together we watched and waited …

Our daughter Jenny sat on one side of the bed and I sat on the other. We held his hands. The curtains dividing the two rooms drawn together. Our two small grandsons came and went quietly taking everything in. The nurse was like an angel of calm. She stood peacefully by ready to reassure and answer our questions. At one stage David stopped breathing and we asked her if he had gone. She thought that he had not, and he breathed again.

The words of my spiritual director came back to me with authority. 'Loving is letting go. The most loving thing you can do is to let David go.' Also the words of Christ to Mary Magdalene in the garden, after he had risen, came to mind. I thought I had let David go with my head and in my heart. But I had not told him. There was one more step to take. I had to tell him in case he could hear, so that he knew that I was not clinging on to him. Jenny moved over to be beside me. She said quietly, 'We'll look after each other Dad'.

This would have warmed David's heart as it did mine. I leaned close and thanked him for so much in halting tones. Then, meaning it, I told him that I was ready to let him go – to the one who loved us more than we loved each other. In a few minutes he died. Jenny and I held each other.

****

It was just past 7 o'clock in the evening. The nurse standing by said that Jenny and I had said the two things that would have comforted and released him more than any other. His spiritual director had said in his final visit: 'He who can say, "In the end, God," has a strength that is impossible to fathom.'[24] I believe that David returned home to God. He had been heading in that direction for some time, and now he was home at last.

At that moment I was given an awareness that his spirit had left his body, free from struggle and pain, and was, in my imagination, soaring high over the Dee Estuary. His body remained, lifeless now. The nurse laid it out with great reverence while we looked on, even talking to him as she went about her work. It was darker now. This was our Good Friday. We were left with David's body and with memories. His spirit was with us.

A while later at that same evening, aware that the family were still around and on the other side of the curtains, I thought again of our two little boys. I did not want them to be confronted with an empty bed without having the opportunity to see their Grandpa's body, now so peaceful, but devoid of life.

Before ringing the funeral directors to remove his body, I checked with Jenny and asked the boys if they wanted to come and see him. After a moment's hesitation, they came up with a will to his bedside. They were face to face with death for the first time and were not afraid. Sad, yes, but not afraid. David's legacy had already begun.

The boys have a firm foundation on which to build for the rest of their lives.

David's body lay still as we sat and let our tears flow and then composed ourselves. Tomorrow we would wake up to a different world. We had come a step nearer to understanding that, as Henri Nouwen puts it, 'The dance of life has its beginnings in grief.'[25]

What made all the difference was that we were all together, sharing the loss and witnessing the peaceful death of someone we loved, in the presence of children, who took everything in their stride. I think we all grew up a little more.

Chapter 15

A New Dawn

Hope is the bird that sings for the dawn, while it is still dark.[26]

I was alone, but not alone. David had left me in the bosom of my family. He had intended to be there for the party and managed it. This had made all the difference. There was a peace in his presence and this had been part of his gift. It was the end, yet not the end. It was the end of our marriage. It was the end of an era. David was beginning a new life. I had to believe that in my end was my beginning too.

My brain went into overdrive. Thoughts that had been partly submerged came to the surface. I was thankful that months earlier we had started to venture into potentially difficult territory together and to look, in advance, at: 'How will you manage?' and 'What about the funeral?'

Although David and I had prepared for this moment as best we could, the sense of being lifted up was extraordinary and beyond words. I was filled with gratitude for our life together and for the wonderful care we had received from so many, including our neighbours, and the NHS in all its forms.

For our own family, in a tiny corner of history and of the world, we first needed to be still and allow the reality of our loss to sink in. After a while we would need to be practical.

The mini-bereavements along the way had given the family, and Jenny and me, the opportunity to let go gradually. When Jenny was nine she and I had given David his episcopal ring to indicate to him that we recognised his calling to be a bishop as well as his calling to be a husband and father. It was an early 'letting go' to his calling to the wider world beyond the family. It always reminded me not to cling to him, but to let him go.

My thoughts in the first quiet moments after David's death included a brief encounter with self-pity. But I had never liked self-pity in others as it seemed like a dead end. Self-pity and sadness are poles apart. I could choose to feel sorrow for myself after such a relatively short time together in retirement. Alternatively, I could take up the challenge to find another way through before self-pity took hold. David, in difficult times, was always ready to move on before a negative attitude got a foothold. I felt his spirit leading the way. His 'Let's get on with it' of four years ago, when he was given the first diagnosis, seemed to indicate the attitude I should take. Self-pity slunk into the shadows and never returned.

But for all the swirling thoughts I knew there was no immediate rush to be practical. We needed a note of tenderness in our thinking. Jenny and I needed to ponder what had just happened, to be sad, naturally, but also to be thankful for David's life, and to talk together.

The family left us to sit quietly to gather our thoughts. I was surprised at how calm I felt. Something told me that David was safe, and released from pain, and from the many invasions of his body over the years. This was comforting. After that letting go moment, I had no desire to cling to his remains, but I needed to stay with his death a while longer. The first stage of letting go had been completed. There was no shock or disbelief, as there had been at the time of the initial diagnosis. David had gone gently, thank God, and he had gone to where he wanted to be.

After a while there was the question of what to do next. How long would we need to stay with David's body? I was clear that he had gone. Should his body lie there for the rest of the night? Was I the one to decide when it should be removed? Who would sign the death certificate? I had not been in this place before. It was new territory.

I was glad to have the family there. They were gentle and respectful, leaving Jenny and me plenty of space to make up our minds what to do. It dawned on me that my caring task was over. A new pathway stretched ahead. Soon we would have to think of funeral plans, but not immediately.

That night Jenny and I rang each of the party guests to tell them that David had died, to save them from hearing the news on the radio or reading it in the paper the following day. I also rang the Chester Diocesan Press Officer with a brief statement of the facts.

After a while Jenny and I felt that the time had come to ring the funeral directors and ask them to come and remove David's body to a Chapel of Rest. It was another letting go moment. The funeral directors were so helpful and gentle in their approach to our questions.

Late that night, two men arrived after the boys had gone to bed. They discreetly removed David's body and placed it in their van. They drove away leaving the bed empty. That night I continued to sleep in the sun-room alongside the empty bed, and I slept peacefully. My sister had put a hot water bottle into my bed.

A new day dawned. It was David's birthday when he would have been seventy-six years old. It was the first day of the rest of my life. Early in the morning, my 6-year-old grandson Stuart came downstairs and slipped into the bed beside me. 'Granny,' he said, 'where has Grandpa gone?' Once again I found that I needed to separate the body from the spirit and gave him an answer, briefly and factually and in two halves. I told him that Grandpa's body had been moved and driven away in a silver-coloured van to the Chapel of Rest so that people who wanted to could visit him. His spirit – the real live Grandpa who lived inside his body – had gone home to God in heaven who made him. Despite the mystery remaining, Stuart seemed quite content. We chatted on under the duvet.

The time had come to think about the funeral plans. David had not left very definite instructions. So we had to use our imaginations, with invaluable help from our rector, Roger Clarke, and from Mark Boyling, who had been one of David's chaplains years ago, and who came to visit us from Carlisle. Quite quickly we decided that as David had been a public figure as well as a private person, we could not hug him to ourselves. For the private person, we decided to hold the funeral at our local church where we had been rooted in retirement, St Bridget's in West Kirby. There we had made many friends and received so much support. I took a lot of advice about the best way to include his public persona in the funeral. We approached various figures from his professional life to ask if they would take part.

After most of the family had departed, Jenny and my sister Evelyn and I remained together for a week, until the funeral. We quickly fused into a harmonious team putting our differing skills to work and creating a rhythm of work and rest to keep us going. Letters and cards of condolence were coming in at the rate of over a hundred a day. Many flowers were delivered. Evelyn sat patiently and methodically for hours, opening and listing every item of mail, and keeping the flowers freshened up. She also doubled up as our housekeeper and my personal minder. Jenny was in effect my personal assistant as we worked together on the funeral plans. She collected the death certificate and was mistress of the computer as the funeral service drafts took shape, and contributors were briefed and kept informed.

I read the many letters in batches when there was a space from the phoning and the funeral planning. The house became a hive of activity, and there were gales of laughter from time to time, mostly initiated by my mischievous sister.

The roller coaster continued. Two days after David's death I experienced chronic leg and foot cramp during the night. It was comforting not to be alone while it gripped me. Later on that second day Archbishop Desmond Tutu phoned from South Africa. He spoke of his respect for David and recalled memories of his anti-apartheid protest, thanking God for his ministry and friendship. He laughed the infectious Tutu laugh, and then asked if he might bless me in Xhosa, his mother tongue, after saying a prayer for us all. Some time later he rang again and left a message on the answerphone. I kept this message for weeks afterwards so that I could listen again. This was part of the tsunami of comfort that washed over us. Flowers kept arriving. I decided to wear black for the funeral to keep things straightforward. My friend Liz went shopping and brought home several suitable outfits for me to try on.

All the people we approached to take part in the funeral agreed to do so, despite busy diaries. On the day, 17 March, our rector Roger Clarke led the service at St Bridget's. The Bishop of Liverpool, James Jones, contributed, and there was an ecumenical element as the Roman Catholic Archbishop Patrick Kelly said some prayers. David's friend Mike Brearley from the world of cricket provided a remembrance, as did his surgeon Carol Makin, who paid tribute to his courage and inspiration. David's spiritual director, Canon Brian McConnell, led the prayers with my spiritual director, the Roman Catholic priest Monsignor John McManus.

Bishop Michael Henshall of Warrington gave the address. He had been David's colleague for twenty years. David's sister, Mary Maxwell, read Psalm 139: 'O Lord, You have searched me and known me … If I ascend into heaven you are there …' His niece, Sarah Maxwell, sang Rutter's Gaelic Blessing, and the St Peter's Singers, of which we had both been members, performed the spiritual, 'Joshua fit the battle of Jericho'. David had loved to sing it with gusto in his bass voice. Professor Ian Tracey, the organist of Liverpool Cathedral, brought his magic touch to the organ at St Bridget's and the instrument sprang to life. The Bishop of Chester, Peter Forster, gave the blessing. It all came together so well.

At the end of the service the family joined the procession. To crown it all, our youngest grandson Gilles, aged four, suddenly stepped out in front leading the way with complete confidence. It brought joy to my heart to walk behind this little boy, with his unselfconscious desire to step out into the future. Afterwards, his 5-year-old brother Stuart said how much he enjoyed the service, 'especially Sarah's singing'.

Sixty people came back to the house for lunch – family and friends from all over the country. That evening we sat thirteen round the table and neighbours generously provided beds and breakfasts for our overflow. March 17th was also Jenny's birthday. I baked her a cake. I wrote in my diary:

> March 17   11.40pm
>
> The funeral is over. David's body has been cremated. A twist in the pit of my stomach reminds me of the finality of today's proceedings. The body that I loved so much and was so thankful for, has gone. Dust to dust. Ashes to ashes …

The family gradually returned to their own homes. David's sister Mary and I were left to claim some calm together.

* * * * *

After the funeral, David's body was cremated at Landican Cemetery and Crematorium. The flag on the Town Hall in Wallasey was lowered half-mast. Six months later his ashes were interred at

Liverpool Cathedral on 23 September and laid under a simple stone slab in the floor engraved with his name and dates. Services of thanksgiving were held in his memory at Liverpool Cathedral, Southwark Cathedral, at Sussex County Cricket Club Ground and in the Mayflower Family Centre in Canning Town, East London.

The letters and cards of condolence kept coming. Within a few weeks nearly a thousand had been put through the letter box. May God bless Ian our postman who carried them all. Two weeks after the funeral my sister-in-law Mary travelled back to Sussex. I was now alone with an open pathway in front of me. I started on the journey by washing bedlinen, shampooing a carpet, and getting out into the garden.

Chapter 16

The Power of Gratitude

Gratitude never faileth:
For gratitude is the herald of faith,
and faith, the harbinger of hope.[27]

The roller coaster had finally come to a halt. I was home alone now. I needed time to reflect, rest and reconnect with friends. I was fortunate in loving our home. David and I had created it together and everywhere I looked there were reminders of him. I was thankful. Not everyone is able to feel that way after the death of a loved one. David's spirit infused and infuses my home, my garden and my relationships. My relationship with Christ is ongoing and brings his promise that I will never be alone. He has left me many signs of his presence. The word comfort means 'with strength', and we only have to look for those signs to be comforted. Then we can go on and be thankful. Gratitude has a power of its own to build instead of to destroy.

Judging by some of the comments I received, there were expectations that I would want to move. I was quite clear that I wanted to stay. This feeling was a gift. I have wonderful neighbours who were quick to welcome me. Jenny saw how content I was and told me never to leave. Her support has been so affirming over the subsequent years.

I was not being allowed to be lonely and I relished this. At the same time I found I was enjoying my solitude, after such a sociable and busy period. The huge pile of condolence letters now presented a challenge. I scooped up the sheaf of mail, and listened to the answerphone messages. I quickly decided that I would answer every letter myself, adding a personal paragraph or sentence at the end of the letter. I would read each letter unhurriedly and answer a specific point made, out of respect for the time and thought that had been taken in writing it. I believed that this would lead me down a positive path and reinforce my belief in the power of gratitude to fend off despair and to bring hope. It would be therapeutic. Best of all it would be a pleasure and not a burden. I was determined to maintain a positive attitude, so it was necessary to develop a feasible strategy.

I was going to try to deal with at least ten letters a day. Two friends offered to address the envelopes for me. Answering the letters was a wonderful and fulfilling exercise which took me to the end of the year. While demanding a good deal of discipline, it helped me to feel connected and caught up in the wave of loving support from so many friends through the positive memories of David that they shared with me.

After forty-eight years of marriage I was a widow. To my surprise I did not feel desperately alone or even deserted. Perhaps that would come later. For the present it felt like a gift. More than four years later I can testify that I have not felt lonely once. This surely is a gift to be received and to be used. Alone, yes: but not isolated or deserted. I have felt among friends.

Owning the label 'widow' felt strange. At first I felt a little disabled as though a limb was missing. But not for long. David had believed in me. He had given me strength and unconditional love. Now I had to believe in myself more than ever and learn a new kind of interdependence.

The word 'widow' held many connotations. I wondered, momentarily, what others would make of it and of me. A few anxious questions surfaced. Would friends change in their attitude towards me? Would some disappear into the shadows? Now that David had gone, would they begin to worry that I would collapse? Who among them still regarded me as a friend? Would our friends turn out to be David's friends after all? Some would, of course. Others would remain in touch. How did I see myself? Was I the deserted one, or was I the one who felt blessed by all those years of building a loving partnership?

I concluded that much would depend on my own effort to maintain the friendships that mattered to me. Quite quickly, I felt a strong compulsion to return to the mainstream and to pick up my life again: life that had necessarily been redirected to caring day and night for my beloved man. I wanted to rejoin my friends in the various groups I belonged to, and to thank them for their support. I had a lengthening list of friends who had been widowed and could learn from them when the time was right. But all in good time.

The flowers and messages of sympathy and goodwill continued to flood in, taking my breath away. Somehow they were saying, 'You'll be OK. We're here if you need us. We love you.' My faith in God was strengthened. His presence was reflected in the people around me. My understanding of the curious words of Christ to his disciples at the Last Supper that he would never leave them, but would die the following day, took on new meaning. It was Christ's spirit that would remain with them. It would be real enough and strong enough to carry them through life's challenges, including struggle and death in the future. It would equip them for their mission to carry on the friendship that Christ had demonstrated. It would also bring them joy.

Friendship was to be the conduit for them: friendship with God, with each other and with themselves. This friendship was to stretch into the nooks and crannies of the world for centuries to come, wherever there was loss and loneliness, disease and poverty. This Holy Spirit was available to all of us for all time. This Spirit of Christ was available for me every day.

Tears would come when I remembered intimate moments. They would come when I remembered David's courage and his patience: when, for example, he had to tuck his syringe driver under his pillow night after night. He knew that when getting up in the night he had to be alert and careful not to pull out the line into his chest and disconnect the appliance. It was a bulky thing, like a small old-fashioned tape recorder or camera on a strap, and he had had to wear it round his neck day and night.

After his ileostomy he had to deal with two fistula bags on his abdomen. He applied himself to new disciplines without fuss until they became an art. Tears of indignation sprang to my eyes when I saw him lying flat with his head wrapped in a mask and strapped to a couch for radiotherapy for his brain. I shared his frustration and sense of helplessness, watching the many abortive attempts to find a vein. His body had become a pincushion. We sighed and sometimes joked together wryly: 'There we go again', as one of his fistula bags leaked once more, and had to be changed. Such recollections bring tears if I choose to revisit them. David's patience and acceptance of suffering moved me and inspired me.

Latterly David wept more easily too. The words of the hymn-writer Brian Wren always moved him to tears with their reference to Christ washing the feet of his disciples.

> We strain to glimpse your mercy seat
> And find you kneeling at our feet.[28]

For me, today, they are tears of enlightenment. They touch the root of faith and the nature of the God we worship.

My tears after David's death were different from any I had experienced before. I think they were tears of love overcoming fear. I was not ashamed of them. I knew they were natural. They felt like a gift. I had to remember that we are all different and grieve in our own different ways.

Many people are fearful of saying or doing anything that might increase the pain of a bereaved person or present themselves with emotion they could not handle. They can sometimes cross the road or avoid saying or doing anything at all in order to save embarrassment. This can leave a person feeling isolated. I was never aware of that happening to me. But I quickly began to realise that I had a part to play in making it easier for people to say hello by making the first move.

I had to be careful not to shed tears indiscriminately as they embarrassed and distressed some people who would react too quickly and give advice – I suspect in order to cheer me up. Trusted friends knew that tears were natural and grief would pass. These friends respected my dignity, believing that I could manage my own emotions. Sometimes they wept with me. But generally they simply sat still without flapping until the tears had passed. While tears of grief are natural, they can cleanse and heal. I could smile at myself through these times because I knew there was hope – hope that life would continue in the face of death. But it is not like this for everyone.

On the day that my sister-in-law Mary left there was a call from the Bishop's office in Liverpool. It was Margaret, Bishop James Jones's personal assistant, asking if he could visit on Good Friday, in a few days time, to talk over plans for the proposed Thanksgiving Service in Liverpool Cathedral. I agreed and contacted Jenny who drafted some thoughts via email for me to edit, ready for our meeting. Bishop James came on Good Friday, bringing a bunch of flowers from the garden at Bishop's Lodge. He was accompanied by the new Precentor of the cathedral, Canon Toby Forward, who would be responsible for the service. Bishop James made it clear that they wanted to do whatever I and the family wanted. He was most helpful and we shared ideas. Although this gave us a free hand, it was clear that we would need to work closely with both diocese and cathedral in order to come to a common mind over the form of worship and other practical considerations. After this meeting, the scale of the task dawned on me. But my fears were gradually subsumed in doing what had to be done. Our imaginations began to work, as Jenny and I decided what we wanted as a family. With the help of two close colleagues who had worked with David, we gradually found the picture coming together in exciting ways.

David's life spread out before us as we recalled his ministry in its various forms over the years. I was clear that he would not have wanted us to be sad, but to move on into a place of thanksgiving to God for the privilege of his calling, and for Christ himself. I was also conscious that as well as parishioners from the diocese, there would be many people coming from a distance who might not have had an opportunity to grieve.

As we worked at the content of the service, and realised the importance of David's calling, a theme emerged. Vocation became a thread in the liturgy and culminated in a moving address by Judge Mark Hedley.

Jenny too was keen that the service should be one not just of thanksgiving, or just of grieving for the loss of someone so inspiring. She thought that with so many people present, we should make the most of the opportunity. We should use it, as David so often did, as a way of encouraging all those who were still actively committed to their own callings, in varied areas of work.

Together with Toby Forward, we decided to start the liturgy with a quiet reflective beginning and move on from there. Thanks to Toby's skill of working on the final draft it all came together. My computer skills had had to be winched up a notch or two, as communicating with diocese, cathedral, family members and contributors took a great deal of time and energy.

Two months later, on 23 May, Liverpool Cathedral was thronged with more than three thousand people from all walks of life. It was a joyful celebration, spanning fifty years and more. Bishop James welcomed the congregation. There were representatives from the diocese and parishes of Liverpool, the main denominations and other faith communities, and the civic authorities. Lord Puttnam spoke for the House of Lords and Johnny Barclay for the world of cricket. St Mary's, Islington, and Southwark Diocese were represented and a coach load of forty people associated with the Mayflower Family Centre in Canning Town came up from the South. The Archbishop of Canterbury, Rowan Williams, gave the blessing.

There were many highlights. David's niece Sarah Maxwell agreed to sing again, as she had at David's funeral. We chose one of his favourite pieces of music, Mozart's 'Exultate Jubilate'. Sarah's beautiful voice resonated through the vast space, touching our spirits with pure joyfulness. Canon Nicholas Frayling[29] read a message from Archbishop Desmond Tutu, and, in his own inimitable way as a friend and colleague and supreme storyteller, had us in fits of laughter over one or two anecdotes at David's expense, lightening the atmosphere.

I had asked Jenny if she felt she could speak for the family. She accepted, and told me that she was doing so because she knew exactly what she wanted to say. It sprang from a particular moment on the day after her father's death. Jenny had been driving back from Birkenhead Town Hall after collecting the death certificate, tears running down her cheeks as she listened to a radio phone-in with Roger Phillips of Radio Merseyside. Local people were ringing in with their moving recollections of David.

She wanted to thank the people of Merseyside for what they had given David. During the Service of Thanksgiving, she told them that he could not have achieved what he did without them. David had been a man who relied on his allies – his friends – a man who had been inspired by his fellow human beings as well as by the love of God. He had been so effective because the relationship had been clearly two-way: a giving and receiving.

I had been keen to include symbols as well as words and music. I had located a young cricketer from Sefton Cricket Club, Peter Kelly, who carried David's cricket bat. His ordination Bible was taken forward by Robbie from the L'Arche Community whom we had met years ago on our first visit. Together these young men carried the symbols and laid them on a table at the front. Many spoke afterwards of being touched by this image.

As we walked out with Professor Ian Tracey playing on the great organ, balloons cascaded down on the worshippers, as they had done eight years before when David had resigned and we had moved on to retirement.

Filled with gratitude after the service, I stood at the back greeting people, which was a heart-warming experience. Someone handed me a large white plastic bag containing something. I was told that it was a photograph for me to keep, but because of the queue of people waiting, I was unable to appreciate the contents at the time. When I opened the bag at home I found that it contained a life-size head and shoulders colour photograph of David, taken at the beginning of our time in Liverpool. It was a living likeness and I was thrilled. But there was no indication of who had given it.

For two years this photograph remained in the hall with other mementos and always with fresh flowers from the garden. It brought comfort and joy and helped me to come to terms with bereavement. I wanted to thank the person who had given it to me and I continued to ask around.

One day I put a notice in the Liverpool diocesan mailing, asking if anyone could shed light on my mystery donor. I received a phone call from a clergywoman who said, 'He lives in my parish!' The mystery was solved. The photographer and his wife came over for a cup of tea and I was able to thank him personally. He has since mounted the photograph on board and it now hangs on the wall, halfway up the stairs, for me to enjoy each time I pass.

Far from making me sad, it has played a huge part in adding to my store of gratitude. I find that tangible things have a place in bereavement as long as they do not become idols. While spiritual gifts are more lasting, all gifts can reflect God's nature and his generosity. Remembering to be thankful is what keeps the connection with the giver, and saves us from taking one another for granted. Giving thanks before meals has gone out of fashion, but it can be a daily reminder of the Giver of Life who sustains us, and it can help to establish a positive habit for when life gets tough.

Chapter 17

Called by Name

When you part from your friend, you grieve not;
For that which you love most in him may be
clearer in his absence, as the mountain to the climber
is clearer from the plain.[30]

Bereavement is challenging. For a married person, it is a time to come to terms with being single again and to rediscover an identity apart from the one to whom one has been joined. This takes time and it does not pay to hurry the process. I came from a large family and I had married young, so it was a new experience to find myself living alone as a single person. Personal friendships made and nurtured over the years have come into their own, as have friendships that we made as a couple. Those connections remain to be continued.

In losing a loving partner, there is a great gap relating to physical contact. It is a time to recognise this and to accept that life will be different. I knew I would miss the closeness David and I had enjoyed over fifty years. I would have to address this loss in my new life and be open to the affection that others might or might not want to offer me. I would have to find a balance that was comfortable.

Informing people of David's death and asking for his name to be deleted from lists was not easy. I felt almost guilty, yet at the same time I knew that this was helping me to face reality. Quite early on I went into David's study to start sorting the contents of his desk. I stayed there too long and after a while I started to feel disturbed and sick. Then the words, 'There's no hurry,' came back into my mind to counsel me. I have found that there is a need to be gentle at such times and pacing is everything. A bull in a china shop only breaks things.

It is sometimes difficult for friends and acquaintances to know what to do or say for fear of upset, and the helps and hindrances vary from person to person. Keeping contact with other people is important and I shall never forget a phone call I received during our Liverpool days when David was in hospital for a hip operation. The surgeon had rung me to say that David had 'put a toe over the touchline'. He had nearly died from a pulmonary embolism. I had kept a candle burning throughout the night.

Knowing that David was in hospital, a priest had rung me. He said, 'I think you must be swamped with calls, and I don't want to be a nuisance, but I'm going to ring you anyway to say that our prayers are with you.' In fact no one had rung that day, which was unusual. I was deeply touched that this man had taken the risk of acting on instinct and had made the phone call. It was a real act of friendship. Ever since, I have done likewise and rung someone who has been on my mind just in case they were feeling alone.

Some expressions from well-wishers crop up fairly often and have given me food for thought. 'Keeping busy then?' is one; 'Look after yourself', another. I have not found 'Keeping busy then?' very helpful. Though well meant, it implies that you may be sitting around with nothing to do and moping, and that you may need a little prod to get going.

'Keeping busy then?' also implies that being still is dangerous and only leads to moroseness, which it can of course if taken to extremes. While understanding that this is said, I believe that there are better ways of greeting a person struggling with loss. Being still to reflect is important from time to time, especially for busy people. A great many people are too busy, and even retired people often speak of being busier than they ever were before. A too-busy person is a restless person. It is a balance that I seek.

It is important to find ways of being comfortable with stillness at any time. 'Look after yourself', on the other hand, is a gentle protective reminder from someone who cares.

One of the most positive and helpful remarks for me in the early days of bereavement was, 'There's no hurry'. It introduced a note of tenderness into the process of dealing with loss and reduced the tension. A simple, 'How's it going?' or 'How are you?' can be all that is needed, especially if the person waits for your reply.

In my garden I have an area which I call the Resting Place. Here I put plants that have bloomed and need to be away from the sun and wind for bit while they 'die down'. This enables them to store energy for another year. Plants can sit out of the limelight and take stock, while others bloom. It is also a place for nurturing new things. Plants, like us, need a rhythm and periods of rest and refreshment.

Now that I was free to design my own life I looked forward to creating a pattern of work and rest that produced maximum energy, but did not send out messages of being too busy for other people. Creating this pattern is an art and needs cultivating. It involves saying 'Yes' and 'No' in the right places.

I had had a good model – years of being married to a man with a full diary, who also believed in aiming to create a good rhythm for day-to-day living. He achieved it often. The secret, for David, lay not only in discipline but also in regular written reviews of his life. This he did with a colleague when at work, and, in retirement, with his spiritual director. I frequently return to a mantra passed on to me by a friend years ago, which she had found helpful:

> To be holy,
> to be really alive, we need
> discipline,
> artistry – and a little foolishness.[31]

I try to practise this now – and I have no trouble with 'a little foolishness', for it comes naturally.

Soon after David's funeral, to steady myself, I made a list of the factors that seemed to be important in maintaining a lively balance of body, mind and spirit. I fixed it onto a kitchen cupboard door as a reminder of the new order. Not in order of priority, it included food (e.g. regular wholesome meals); fresh air and exercise (e.g. walking and gardening); duty and discipline (e.g. maintenance and desk); pleasure and creativity (e.g. hobbies, culture and enter-tainment); family and friends (e.g. keep in touch); outreach and care (e.g. community and church involvement); rest (an hour a day); spiritual direction (e.g. regular review and accountability); and worship/devotion (alone and in church). This seemed to cover most eventualities. Four to five years later the list is still there and has served me well. I wanted to be like an elastic band that retained its elasticity: able to move in and out, capable of being stretched from time to time but also able to relax.

Alongside all the sorting out, attending thanksgiving services and answering the condolence letters, I was developing a new identity. Saying 'I' instead of 'we' felt awkward and slightly self-centred. But I had to get used to it.

An unexpected invitation

Three weeks after the funeral I received an unexpected invitation. Would I be willing to open the Dee Artists' Art Exhibition? David and I had been members of the Dee Artists' Group. I had been wondering what else life might have in store, and I had hopes of getting started with the book that I had been planning to write just before David's original diagnosis.

On receiving the invitation, my first reactions were of surprise and delight that I had been approached. Fatigue comes with bereavement and my energy levels were low. This invitation stirred something deep within, motivating me to stand up, join the community and start living my own life again. I thought of Mary Magdalene in the garden of Gethsemane, distraught, exhausted and confused after witnessing the crucifixion of someone she valued and loved. Confronted by Christ after his resurrection, and thinking him to be the gardener, her sore eyes were opened. What liberated her and confirmed her identity was to hear her name called. 'Mary,' he said, and, 'Don't cling to me ...', and 'Go ...'. Christ had work for her to do and he gave her the strength for the task. She had not been abandoned after all. She ran to join the others, to share her news.

The invitation from the Dee Artists' Group felt a bit similar. Someone was calling me by name to get out there and join in. Although widowed, it appeared I still had something to offer, even at this early stage. I agreed to do it. This helped me to hold up my head and make the effort to go forward a little further. Later on there were other interesting and challenging invitations. Life began to look exciting.

The months flew by. I attended the other thanksgiving services, except for the one at Southwark Cathedral at which Jenny represented us. The Thanksgiving Service on the turf of the Sussex County Cricket Club Ground in Hove took place in hot sunshine. The journey had been a challenge as I had chosen to drive to Sussex – the first long drive alone since David's death. We had shared the driving when he was well. David had mostly done our navigating when we travelled together. He relished it. But I was not good with maps and it took a long time to work out a route to Sussex, sometimes needing to turn the map upside down to get my bearings. The time and nervous energy spent on this was more than I was willing to spend. I wanted to enjoy the drive and save my energy for meeting people.

I learnt a useful lesson which was to acknowledge my limits. I bought a navigation system which was a triumph. Acknowledging limits is important for an ageing person, as the physical boundaries draw in. There is life within the new confines and there are risks to be taken and courage to find.

After a week in Sussex, visiting friends and relatives in eleven different places, together with attending the service at the Sussex County Cricket Club ground, I returned home – 680 miles later. I felt fresh and was grateful for yet another gift, this time of renewed confidence in driving across the country. I shall never forget the generous welcome from the cricket fraternity, both in Sussex and at Lords later on. I have continued to visit Sussex County Cricket Club each year. To keep a link with David they graciously made me a Vice-President.

Summer 2005 gave way to autumn and Christmas was on the horizon. David and I had always written a newsletter over the years, to enclose in a Christmas card. It had been thematic, reflective and informative, rather than being just a list of family doings.

The feedback was such that we continued to do this in retirement in a careful unhurried ritual so that we did not take our friends for granted. I would write the letter and David would edit it. Until we ventured into the world of computers, one of us would address the envelopes while the other wrote the name on the card. We would share the signing, and the stamping, adding a personal note when appropriate. This enabled us to sit unhurriedly with each person, as it were, and recall them, having their newsletters to us at hand. It became an important connecting link with friends from the past, and with family. It has maintained a closeness that is real and beyond measure. Throughout the year, we would follow a practice of Bishop Mervyn Stockwood and take four or five Christmas cards from the heap each day during our prayer time, and remember the senders with thankfulness.

A bishop has one day off a week and holidays, but usually no weekends. This puts a limit on the time that can be spent with friends in a leisurely fashion, especially if they are scattered. Keeping in touch in this way was important to us over the years. It has proved to be a blessing.

Christmas 2005 was a special time. The family joined me. Our memories of David's last Christmas were good because he had been able to join in the fun, though it was tinged with sadness. For me, the best Christmas present for 2005 came from Radio Three. They did a most courageous thing and broadcast ten whole days and nights of the music of J. S. Bach. I have been a Bach fan since the age of fourteen when witnessing Sir Malcolm Sargent conducting a Bach/Handel concert in the Royal Albert Hall. I had gone with my father. The Radio Three Christmas broadcasts were a taste of heaven. I sang and danced my way through writing cards, cooking and wrapping presents. In my joy and gratitude for such a Christmas gift, I was among the many people who emailed Radio Three to thank them.

I believe David rejoiced with me. Mozart was his favourite composer, but he confessed latterly to falling for Bach as well. Music has a way of touching those soul places of loss with consummate healing. Weeping may endure for a night, but joy comes in the morning, says the psalmist.

Christmas cards came pouring in as before, only this time, my name was alone on the envelope. The year 2006 dawned. I had survived so far and was among friends. The wheels of a brand new roller-coaster ride were beginning to turn.

Chapter 18

A Touching Place

I began to see prayer more as a friendship than a rigorous discipline. It started to become more of a relationship and less of a performance.[32]

Stepping into the new year of 2006 I rattled along the tracks, delighting in the family, and in the loyalty and compassion of so many friends. All this augured well for the future and I looked forward to my new life, and to the challenge of developing a new kind of interdependence. I had to reach out. I also had to have the grace to take the hands that were reaching out to me.

I needed to return to my touchstone regularly. A touchstone was a small dark tablet of stone used, centuries ago, to authenticate gold and silver and to test forgeries. My touchstone was and is Christ, underpinning everything. This is a place where I can and must be truly myself and know that I am loved unconditionally. At the same time I had to remember, like Mary Magdalene in the garden, that I was not meant to cling to Christ, or to David, or to the past. I had to move out into the new life that was being both commissioned and offered.

In returning again and again to Christ our touchstone, we are able to become more authentic human beings. He was fierce in his condemnation of hypocrisy, especially among religious people. He wanted the real thing. Authenticity needs to be the mark of a Christian.

A sense of identity can suffer a few knocks during bereavement. I found that it was important to be honest and to keep in touch with those I trusted and who knew me best. David's question, 'What will you do when I've gone?', would need answering. The months running up to Christmas had been exceptionally demanding because of the usual preparations and several thanksgiving services, and the letters to be answered. Other memorials to David were being planned and I was invited to contribute in one way or another. This meant owning that part of who I was, was still attached to him. That felt reasonably straightforward. The challenge to strike out on my own with fresh goals remained.

Our family Christmas had gone well, but flu struck after the festivities, when my immune system was low. February turned to March. It snowed on my birthday, 4 March. On the doorstep appeared two neighbours, well wrapped up and bearing a homemade birthday cake. It turned out to be one of the happiest birthdays I can remember.

The following day was the first anniversary of David's death and we had a small private Service of Thanksgiving and remembrance in our church, attended by a few local friends.

The snow melted and spring arrived. The garden sprang to life. Snowdrops gave way to daffodils and primroses and the trees and shrubs put on their best green apparel. Life looked good and I was ready to get on with it.

Then one morning, after a shower, I discovered a small lump in my breast. I decided to leave it for a week before contacting the doctor. It did not subside. My doctor referred me to a consultant surgeon who, on 21 March, examined me and invited me to sit down. 'My dear,' he said kindly, but very directly, 'you have breast cancer. You will need surgery.'

After an initial pause for me to take it in, he said, 'I could do you tomorrow. How do feel about that?' It was like two pistol shots, one after the other. But it was not the first time I had faced a cancer diagnosis and I realised that speed was the best policy. The surgeon's offer was a gift. My brain went into overdrive, and was beginning to sort out my priorities. I asked for a few minutes alone to absorb the shock and to ring my daughter before responding to his offer. It was early morning and the surgeon said he could wait until 5 p.m. that day for my reply, but that I would need to undergo various tests.

A nurse showed me to a small side room to gather myself. Tears were shed and quickly wiped away. I rang Jenny in London and was deeply touched by her instant response: 'I'll come up as soon as I can.'

With Jenny's backing I decided to go ahead with surgery the following day, as there was obviously no time to lose. Her husband Donald took responsibility for the two boys and Jenny caught the next train to Liverpool. There was nothing else in my diary for that day except my monthly appointment with Father John in the late afternoon. This was remarkable timing.

Tests were done and I was preparing to go home. I rang Father John to tell him the news and to say that I would be late. He insisted on being at my home on my return and we were able to sit quietly in God's presence and absorb the shock, talking when we felt like it. This was balm indeed. The jerks of the roller-coaster ride settled down. I felt secure and well supported and went to pack a bag, prepared for the next twist and turn in the journey.

The sensitivity and readiness of Jenny to come to my side, and Father John's willingness to be there after a testing day, gave me strength and resolve to move on. There was no time for self-pity or for anger. This swift action on the part of everyone to come alongside was the friendship of Christ personified. Too much time on our hands might have given way to anxiety, self-indulgent licking of wounds and introspection. I could only give thanks that help and support was so readily available, and my part was to get on with it. In my book of meditations and prayers were the words, 'and Jesus reached out his hand and touched the leper'. I wrote in pencil alongside, 'Jesus touched me.'

On the day of the operation, a further entry reads, '22 March 2006 – grateful for the gift of life.' There is power in gratitude. All this, I am sure, helped to set the tone for my attitude to the unwelcome news and gave me courage.

It was perhaps a coincidence that my daily reading for the morning of 22 March began with a prayer by Frank Topping:

> Lord, you came to give us life,
> and life that was more abundant.
> Help me not to run away from life
> but to follow your spirit,
> to accept the thorn as well as the flower,
> and to be grateful for the gift of life.[33]

The surgeon performed a lumpectomy to remove the tumour, some lymph nodes and surrounding tissue. He told me that he had 'got it all'. Extensive internal bleeding delayed my return home, but only by one day. Jenny was with me and after a few days she was able to return to her family. Neighbours took over in keeping an eye on me. One even stayed overnight. Others offered to shop or prepare food and I was touched by the level of care.

I had been informed that daily radiotherapy would follow. A little later I was able to undertake the twenty-minute drive through the countryside to the hospital. It was a beautiful early summer. The hedges had blossomed, inspiring me as I drove in the early morning sunshine, thanking God that I was alive and ready for adventure. It was a well-worn route.

In April I received a letter from the Bishop of Chester which took me by surprise. Would I consider conducting the ordination retreat in July for the men and women to be ordained priest? And would I be willing to preach in the cathedral at the ordination service? This invitation shook me to my foundations. In the circumstances it was out of the question – or so I thought. I asked for time to consider. I had already booked into a local retreat house for a brief period of personal reflection so I took the invitation with me to decide what to do. There were questions to answer. Did I want to do it? Could I do it? Had I enough experience to give me the confidence to try? Did I feel called to do it?

Deep down I wanted to do this. It excited me. But my motivation was quickly threatened by a feeling of inadequacy. July seemed rather close. I had spoken to a variety of groups, and had taken several retreats in the past, but those seemed aeons away then because I had been concentrating on caring for David and my mother for several years.

The thought that I could minister to priests seemed to be the wrong way round. And yet there was a sense of calling – but that was something that needed testing. I consulted several people whom I trusted to tell me the truth. They encouraged me to 'go for it'.

But I would have been undergoing radiotherapy and had no idea how this would affect me. I decided that I would have to refuse as I was not sure that I would have the energy or the time to prepare.

Sitting down to answer the bishop, I reread his letter. In the shock of the moment I had misread the date. The invitation was for

July 2007, a year later. There seemed to be no excuse for dodging the challenge. I remembered my original sense of motivation and accepted, in the faith that I would be alive and well in a year's time.

July 2007 arrived. Radiotherapy was well behind me and I was in good health. With months of preparation under my belt, I jumped in the deep end. I retreated for two days with fifteen candidates for ordination. My theme was 'The Friendship of Christ' and on the chapel steps I placed a small model of Stephen Broadbent's sculpture *The Water of Life*, depicting Christ's meeting with the Samaritan woman at the well.

This remarkable sculpture spoke volumes to me and continues to do so. It portrays the giving and receiving of thirst-quenching, life-giving water. Humanity and divinity combine in mutual respect. Ordinary human need becomes a channel for healing and transformation. This is pure love. Stephen Broadbent's sculpture was our icon for the retreat. It reflected so much of what David and I had experienced in the months and years of facing vulnerability together.

The retreat was one of the most demanding, yet rewarding experiences of my life. I received so much in the giving of it.

The healing affirmative touch of the Bishop's invitation in 2005 had provided me with an alternative focus, something completely apart from cancer management. It had ensured that I re-entered the mainstream of life as a single person, stretching me just enough, enabling me to grow a little more, and backed by the prayers of friends. The Bishop's faith in me helped me to have confidence in myself, as I took my first steps into a new life. Other invitations arrived. I was asked to write, to broadcast and to open events. At present, my X-rays show no sign of recurring cancer.

There were other touches that surprised and delighted me. Offers of hospitality were heart-warming. One friend told me that an invitation to stay meant a lot when she had just lost her husband. Several good friends invited me to stay with them for a couple of nights. One person, in the Lake District, had travelled her own journey of loss some time ago. She created slow relaxing mornings for us both by bringing me breakfast in bed, while she had hers in her room. This friend knew about cherishing. A wonderful peace came over her house, which brought healing in my bereavement. We balanced the silence by talking and relaxing together later over her delicious homemade food.

At times I felt that I had to set the pace with people I did not know well, and make the first move. I had to judge what was appropriate and acceptable each time. Some people are unsure how to approach a recently bereaved person and hold back. Others instinctively open their arms in welcome and affection. The embraces of family and grandchildren are precious and never to be taken for granted. I have been greeted with affection by so many that I need not have worried. A good firm handshake or a touch on the arm are still gifts when hugs seem awkward.

Letters and cards, flowers, music and books all have a part to play. I have even hugged myself, and why not? Someone sent an email entitled 'Just waving' and I waved back. This kept us connected to one another. All I had to do was to receive the affection, be thankful and allow it to spill out to others.

Inevitably there are gaps. I have heard bitter comments from some who feel that they have been abandoned by people they thought were their friends. But people have their reasons for stepping back from relationships that once seemed close. I felt that it was my responsibility to maintain friendships that mean a lot and to let go with care when they fade. We live in a throw-away society and in the same way we can drop relationships, sometimes at our peril. Friends are our lifeblood. They are worth nurturing. Friends can keep an eye on each other.

When David and I moved into retirement, we had wanted a garden. Our new house had a wall of old conifers and shrubs along the front, shutting out light and fencing off the people who walked by on the pavement outside. We stripped out everything except an old apple tree that had been reaching for the light for many years, and was squeezed by the conifers on either side. The border has been replanted with sweet-smelling and colourful shrubs and plants that can be enjoyed by those on both sides of the boundary. I took my secateurs to the gnarled old apple tree. It now has a new life and, like Abraham's Sarah, has even produced little apples late in its life. I can see people walking to and fro and they can see me. Sometimes they wave as they pass and I wave back.

We had designed a garden for others, as well as for ourselves. There are generous expressions of appreciation which delight me.

They motivate me to keep the garden trim and interesting. The connection with others is maintained without us living in each other's pockets. A feeling of family grows in a neighbourhood. We get to know one another's names and cease to become strangers. As Desmond Tutu has often been heard to say, 'We are family'. He goes on to explain another South African word – 'ubuntu' – which means, 'I am because you are.' He says, ' Ubuntu speaks particularly about the fact that you can't exist as a human being in isolation. It speaks about our interconnectedness. You can't be human all by yourself, and when you have this quality – Ubuntu – you are known for your generosity.'[34]

Without one another, we are both nothing and useless in the long run. This is especially true of the experience of belonging to a church. This is another family. At best it is one of the places where faith is fed and where we can lift our hearts and minds to worship the one who is greater: to God himself. It is here that we can enjoy the friendship and fellowship of other human beings who struggle with the issues of life and death and who are there for one another, and also reach out to others. It is also, or should be, a place where all are welcome, including the stranger.

This has been encapsulated in a story I heard from a priest friend who visited Kabul while working on a project for the then Bishop of Pakistan. He went for a walk and encountered something which touched him deeply. He told it like this:

> An elderly man was seated among the rubble – and then I saw it was a particular pile of stones made in a certain way. It was the grave of his son, victim of a recent shelling. He was still and silent in his grief. I crouched down beside him and whispered 'salaam alaikum'. We did not speak much – he did not want to, and my knowledge of Dari was unequal to the situation. But he did hold my hand and beckoned me to stay. We looked at each other. For some moments, we met, person to person, eye to eye, and I was humbled at the honesty of his gaze and his acceptance of the stranger who came at such a moment. I was there for board meetings to plan projects, but here was the starting point: if we cannot meet eye to eye, offering our very selves for that moment, what use were our plans?

This is the essence of real meeting. That the elderly man held out his hand from the heart of his grief is the grace of God in action. The two men, strangers to one another, became acquainted and then became friends. Their lives had touched and been enriched.

We need to return often to Christ our touchstone for refreshment and renewal, and to remember how much we are loved. He is our model. This can save us from play-acting and becoming fakes or hypocrites.

Christ of course cannot be confined to church and our faith home cannot be taken for granted. Our authenticity will depend on how willing we are to meet Christ face to face and eye to eye every day in each person we meet. Much will depend on the image we hold of God. We are reminded again that 'God is friendship'. We see him through the life of Christ and through his faithful followers, since that last supper when he called his disciples to move from being servants into the new relationship of being his friends.

We can run into difficulties because of wanting to be perfect. We are exhorted to be perfect, but not all at once. Other people sometimes expect us to be perfect and to set an example. They quickly become disillusioned when they see that we are just like them, and fail to live up to our standards all the time. This expectation of perfection is a snare and can drive us to pretend and to act a part, out of fear of being rejected. It jars to witness someone smiling with their lips, but not with their eyes. We need to be authentic.

One of the most effective and powerful touching places is prayer. It is the language that connects us to God and to one another in a threefold chord. Prayer can be the vehicle of our heart's innermost longings. During the most testing times of caring for David, I would feel lifted on a tangible wave of peace. I knew that people were praying for us. Just knowing that was enough to bring the strength and endurance that was needed for us both. I could return to this touching place in the most testing of times and know that I was not alone. To know that we are not alone in our struggles makes all the difference in the world. This source of strength and companionship is a great gift and one that I hope I never take for granted as I move towards my own death and final homecoming to God.

Chapter 19

Coming Home

Home is where one starts from.[35]

Coming home has always been a pleasure. I love my home. It is where I belong, and a base where I can relax and be myself. Ideally it is not just a house, but an atmosphere and a place where there is love, given and received. Coming home to someone we love is a special joy. I like to think that heaven will be something like this. The Bible tells us that there will be no more pain and no more tears there. It will be a place where the broken are made whole and the sick are healed. Home is where God is, and coming home to God will be like coming home to someone who loves us.

But much depends on the image of God that we have. Do we imagine meeting an old friend, or perhaps a stranger, or worse, a merciless judge? I see God as a faithful friend. I believe there are glimpses of heaven now, in our everyday lives. For me these glimpses can be seen in acts of kindness, in the laughter of little children, in a piece of music, in the joy of seeing the first peony bloom, and so much more. The key is to keep looking. The earth is full of good things, alongside the death and destruction we read and hear about in the daily news. The more we look for beauty and goodness in one another and in creation, the more we shall see. We will find that we are overwhelmed with joy day by day. Then it becomes natural to be thankful, and to say so to the Creator himself, in worship.

Gratitude is a powerful tool against the ravages of despair. Well before David's illness I was sent a postcard with the quotation, 'Gratitude never faileth: for gratitude is the herald of faith, and faith, the harbinger of hope.' I have not been able to find the source. I found that these words needed to be read slowly, pausing at each phrase, to let the meaning take root. After a while I came to see that an act of gratitude not only encourages faith, but is directly related to hope, and therefore to fending off despair.

That quotation inspired me to practise gratitude for a while. I began consciously to look for things to be thankful for: the everyday things we take for granted. Soon it became a habit and the list grew longer each day. I believe this was part of my preparation for what lay ahead. During David's illness and dying this habit played a major part in keeping my spirits up during some exhausting and worrying times. It had become part of me.

In bereavement too gratitude has been a powerful tool. It has helped me to look up and away from myself. I have received so much practical faithful love, and creation is bursting with gifts. My job is now to receive these gifts graciously, and then, hopefully, the sum of them will spill over to others in unselfconscious ways. This is what happens so often in the hospice movement. Many of the volunteers give their time out of gratitude for the care that they witnessed during a family member's illness and subsequent death.

Sister Frances Dominica, the founder of Helen House, the children's hospice in Oxford, reminds us:

> We can't change the world, but actually, in very small ways
> we can change the world, because we can make a
> difference in our lives, maybe to one person, but a
> profound difference; just by coming alongside, by walking
> a bit of the journey with them, not having the answers, but
> having the courage to stay in the unknowing with them.
> That's what friendship is I think.

There are many glimpses of heaven to be found in the hospice movement. In our experience, nurses, doctors and volunteers alike worked as a team with healing in mind. It was in their eye contact, as we checked in and when they called us by our names. Their smile of welcome and their sense of calm, despite their own busyness, reassured us. The way they made the bed with care, and the outstretched helping hand or offered arm spoke volumes. They enabled us to feel that David was not just an NHS number, but a human being with feelings. I was not just someone to be tolerated, but instead I was treated as part of the team. Their careful explanation of procedures and treatments gave us under-standing. There was gentleness in the way dressings were changed. Their watchfulness and their laughter made us feel secure. They appeared to have time to listen and to help us not to feel abandoned or alone, and we were even touched by their tears! They truly suffered with us. They also rejoiced with us. Humanity was allowed to shine through the professionalism. The hospice became a home from home.

All this and much more I witnessed as a carer. Hospice care begins to paint a picture of heaven as I believe it to be. A godly empathy neither deserts nor dominates. But it is always 'there', seeking to bring dignity and comfort, with a listening sensitivity. It brings love without sentimentality, and good practice in all its forms. The hospice movement is showing us how to 'do' friend-ship and how to provide the best professional help for those facing the end of their lives. This level of care need not be confined to hospices, but we can seek to learn from them in order to practise it in our day-to-day relationships. It is about respecting one another. I believe it could change the world.

Now that David has gone on ahead, I come home to a place that is full of memories. I am learning to live with myself in a new way and I know that I am not alone. Being over seventy I am in 'bonus time'. I need to attend to preparing for my own death: to be practical and to treasure my friends and family. I will return to the one who made me and loved me enough to give his life for me, and who never left me alone. I like to think that returning to God will mean that I will be reunited with David in some mysterious way and with all those I have known and loved who have gone before me. All the same I am content to live with the mystery.

Though his body is in ashes under the cathedral floor, David's spirit remains as a real presence that is not just sentimental mem-ories. His essence infuses my home and thinking. Christ promised never to leave his disciples yet died the following day. His essence too infuses our lives. There is truth in the words of the fourth-century St John Chrysostom, which were sent to me soon after David's death: 'He whom we love and lose is no longer where he was before. He is now wherever we are.'

If heaven is like coming home, then some of the ingredients are worth considering. Home is both a place and a relationship. For

David and me, home was the place that we created and designed together. It was not just the colours, the design and the objects. Home was the place where we learned to relate to each other in love and trust, and to relate to all who passed across our threshold. Here we learned to be and to say sorry and to forgive and to be forgiven. It was the place in which we learned about being a family. We could make mistakes and pick ourselves up again and be accepted. It was a place where we recognised the presence of the God of love at all times, including the difficult and testing ones. Home was also open to others. It was a place of hospitality where we loved to eat and drink with friends.

It is good to feel at home with someone. A major factor in being able to 'let go' in death is the extent to which we have felt at home with God in everyday life and looking for facets of his character in every person and in ordinary things. If we have learnt to feel at home with God, he will not feel such a stranger when the time comes to meet him in death. In the words of the Roman Catholic priest Daniel O'Leary, 'God's face is in every face, a God who comes to us disguised as life.' Looking for him, and learning to be at home with one another in life is the task and the training ground for our dying. Our pattern is Christ.

I know how blessed I still am to enjoy coming home. It is remarkable to me that, having lost my best friend and husband of nearly fifty years, I have not felt uncomfortably lonely. I know that there is always something I can do to prevent loneliness before it takes root. There is a difference between solitude and loneliness and I enjoy a certain amount of solitude. I have had to learn to be friends with myself in bereavement, as well as with others, and with God. Faithful friendship is life-giving. It is in relationships that God can be encountered most tellingly. In the words of Canon Eric James, 'it's in and through my friends that I think I have learnt, and still do learn, most about God, and receive most from him.'[36] That has been true for me.

But for friendship to thrive it needs to be two-way. Effort and sacrifice is involved in keeping a relationship alive. One of the major challenges for me during David's decline was to keep in touch with those who enquired, keeping them informed of his progress. It was equally challenging to find the time to acknowledge and keep up with post, emails and telephone messages. The act of thanking people kept the door open, through which the love and prayers of so many could flow. Good communication was vital. Once again gratitude worked its power to heal and to bring hope.

When Christ met the woman of Samaria at the well, divinity and humanity met eye to eye, person to person. Christ and the woman exchanged gifts that refreshed and renewed them both in a holy friendship. A simple cup of water made all the difference to each person. Christ departed, physically refreshed from the human encounter and her cup of water. She in turn went forward refreshed in spirit, by the living water of unconditional pure love offered and received from the Son of God. She had also received the respect of a man from another culture. The story of the woman at the well inspires me to remember to nurture my humanity and divinity each day. It prompts me to be still before God with gratitude, and to bring my needs and the needs of others in prayer, and then to act on them where possible. We were designed for the benefit of one another in an unbroken threefold cord.

Many of us are afraid of dying and of talking about dying. We have no knowledge of the way we will die, and have only hints of what life after death will be like. It is an unknown mystery. Perhaps we have been involved with difficult deaths or heard stories second hand, so we shy away from looking at it and talking about it, in case we are taken unawares; in case we are infected by it before we are ready. But this is to avoid the inevitable and to create anxieties that may revisit us repeatedly until the end. It is helpful to be ready.

Living with dying can be like mountaineering. Explorers do not venture out alone, but have a team behind them. Having lost three close members of his family to cancer, Sir Ranulph Fiennes finally scaled the highest mountain in 2009 at his third attempt. This time he was sixty-five years old. He said that the way for him to get to the top was to 'plod on for ever'. He suffers from vertigo and said to himself, 'Don't look down.' In the same way my mother would say when the going was tough, 'You just put one foot in front of another.' What endurance and courage with which to inspire us! Sir Ranulph offers excellent directions for us to follow if we want to die well: 'Plod on' and 'Don't look down!'

Like explorers and adventurers, we need to prepare carefully for death. Living with David's dying was certainly an adventure. We both felt like explorers in a new world which was full of surprises, both welcome and unwelcome. This new world was dangerous and called for courage. It was distressing and comfort was needed. Emotional and physical exhaustion took its toll. It was frightening, yet love came to our rescue. Plodding on with people for company, and resisting the urge to look down, was certainly a major part of the action. We knew where we were heading.

But we were surprised by joy so often in the little things. Each time we set off for the hospital for a consultation, a treatment, an X-ray, or for David to be admitted for pain relief or surgery, not knowing what was in store, we saw the trip as an adventure, a foray into the unknown. We had to learn to live with mystery. But we were ready for surprises and we had each other. Family, friends and the NHS became our team. We also shared a faith in God who is there both in the present moment and beyond. A great deal of the journey involved breaking new ground.

But it was an adventure that we entered into knowing that, as David put it at the time of his first diagnosis, 'I've got to die of something.' The secret was to look for ways of living life to the full alongside the dying. After each visit to hospital we came home and put the kettle on. We made some tea and relaxed. Coming home was a taste of heaven each time. Towards the end of his life, while in the hospice, David became unsettled. He said that he wanted to go home. That was where he wanted to die.

There is an apparent contradiction for some of us who love life and are not ready to die yet. Towards the end of his life David said something which I recorded in my journal, and which illustrates the problem. I had been getting very tired and needed some respite from the disturbed nights and 24-hour care of the last few years in order to survive. Reluctantly I was going to have to accept more help from the NHS in my care of David. I wrote down some of what was involved, so that I could break it up into sections and see what I would gradually have to hand over to the nurses, and what would be left for me still to do. For instance, two people would eventually be needed to help David in and out of the bath. 'We've come to wash the bishop!' said the two auxiliary nurses with a big smile as they stood on the doorstep one morning.

I shared my written thoughts with David. My journal records the following response from him.

> 17/12/04
> 'Wow! What a palaver!'
> 'Which palaver did you mean?' I said.
> 'Dying slowly,' he said.
> 'Yes!' I said. 'But you are still alive! – and I'm glad,' I said.
> 'Yes,' he said. 'I want to live.'

Living with dying is a palaver. Until the final weariness sets in, there is a lot of living to do within the changing boundaries. David was good at that.

The will to live is a gift. I would certainly want to die living as fully as possible. But we cannot know exactly how or when our dying will happen. We can only prepare as best we can, continue to be grateful for life and then get on with living together in the friendship of Christ until it is time to go home.

Richard Gillard's hymn says it all:

> Brother, sister, let me serve you,
> Let me be as Christ to you:
> Pray that I may have the grace to
> Let you be my servant too.
>
> I will hold the Christlight for you
> In the night-time of your fear;
> I will hold my hand out to you,
> Speak the peace you long to hear.
>
> I will weep when you are weeping;
> When you laugh, I'll laugh with you.
> I will share your joy and sorrow
> Till we've see the journey through.
>
> When we sing to God in heaven,
> We shall find such harmony,
> Born of all we've known together,
> Of Christ's love and agony.

Appendix 1

Poem

Prayer/poem composed before addressing the Chester Time Out Conference for Clergy Spouses, and after David's return from hospital.

Dear Lord,

I'm all of a twitter this morning,
My head is in a flat spin;
The women are coming tomorrow
For some time-out together, but no gin.

I'm supposed to be speaking tomorrow,
With talks all well prepared;
But honestly, Lord, there's one still to write
And concentration has disappeared.

I must iron David's trousers,
He's off to the doctor today.
The soup that he made leapt all over them
During lunch on our laps yesterday.

I must make the bed, wash my hair and have breakfast;
And see Peter who's coming to dig.
I must go to the loft for a suitcase
To pack a few things in a bag.

I must clear up the spare room for Hazel,
My sister who's coming to stay,
And make sure there's food for the patient,
And washing's done b'fore going away.

We're off to see the oncologist
In an hour or two's time you see,
And we're wondering what he will tell us
And what changes he will decree.

How will D take to chemo?
And what about holiday plans?
What about seeing the grandchildren?
And what's round the corner for us grans?

I was all of a twitter this morning,
My head was in a flat spin;
But thank you for listening: I feel better already.
Now talk to me just for a min.

My Friend replied,

Sit still, my dear daughter, beside me,
And see how the matter will pass.
I am here in the mess and the muddle
Beside you, from first until last.

I am here in the fog and confusion,
I am listening to every word.
Sit quietly here and trust me
That all will be well: I am Lord.

What matters is in the real meeting
Of genuine human encounter;
Not polished performance, or neat briefing;
Take courage. Be honest. Go well.

I am here, and there, and will never
Forsake or leave you alone.
I am there in the others. I am there in creation,
I am there in the mist and the fog.

I am here with you as you are girl,
I will be there when you get onto your feet.
You've done your best. I'll do the rest.
Trust me; you're all in for a treat.

You're never alone, you can do it;
Use your gifts, you're among friends.
They know about life and its muddles,
And I know, and love never ends.

Be a channel through which love can flow,
My love that'll never abandon;
It brings healing and joy in abundance
And solid foundations to stand on.

Today is the one to live fully,
Tomorrow is only a dream.
Already I've been in tomorrow,
And have prepared for all that's unseen.

So live now, love now and risk.
The fog and the mist will part.
Do as I say, and you'll find me
In the others, and in your own heart.

Appendix 2

A Letter to Friends

Towards the end of completing this book the telephone rang. Two long-term friends in their eighties had been thinking about preparing themselves for their end-times. They wondered if I could set down some of what helped David and me to do that, to get them started. Feeling so privileged, it was a request I could not refuse. But as I was deep into the last stages of producing my manuscript for the publisher, I said I would willingly try, but it would have to be in the form of a long letter and unedited. I spent the next day producing the following personal letter which they generously said they found helpful.

It was suggested that I should include it here. Ted and Audrey have given their permission. Although it contains repetition of material in the book, and has not been tidied up, they and I hope that it may help someone else to take a step towards being prepared for death and dying in a way that brings more reassurance and freedom to live life as fully as possible.

****

My dears Ted and Audrey,

First, thank you for the privilege of sharing some of our end-times journey with you.

I have been thinking and praying my way to this moment. All sorts of thoughts popped up into my head while you were talking and since, so I have decided to write you a long letter without spending too much time editing it. It will be 'top-of-head' thinking, and with little finesse! It is Not offered as Advice, but rather a sharing. Take it or leave it.

There are various principles that David and I observed during our journey – not always adhered to … but mostly.

The Colours and Palette of our Loving and Preparation for The End-Times

Live in the Present Moment and hallow it. Don't entertain the 'What if's' for too long. Stop if it gets painful and return later at a better time of day. 'Tomorrow never comes'!

Create home as a place of peace, free from complaints, loud noises and panics! Make a friend and servant of the telephone; i.e. control the answer-phone.

Don't patronise or boss the patient; bolster his will (to live or die); be gentle; be ready to talk.

Look for the gifts your loved one has to offer and be thankful.

Keep close; communicate carefully, using the mobile phone when out if necessary, to minimise anxiety and the fear of being left alone.

Create a safe place (i.e. a spiritual director or soul friend) to lay down the heavier burdens and to keep God in focus; keep touching base with Christ – arrow prayers …

Keep in regular and close touch with family members.

Keep in touch with friends, including church and Bishop Peter (for D and G only).

Keep in touch with neighbours.

Take offers of help seriously and take them up when possible.

Welcome visitors; but don't let them tire the patient …

When applicable, respect the Press, but seek help from a professional when preparing statements.

Retain intimacy together within new boundaries.

Remember the therapeutic qualities of fresh air.

Keep up singing and gardening; homecooking.

Don't be ashamed to rest – I would sometimes lie down on the floor for five minutes and relax.

Keep thanking and praising for what we have.

My 'mantra' has been one that you sent me years ago:

To be Holy,

To be really Alive

we need Discipline

    Artistry

       and

A little Foolishness (Hurray!)

This has turned into a mini-book in itself. Please forgive me for not editing it.

1. Everyone is different. Treat the counselling formulas with a pinch of salt. So know yourself and your limits and then live up to the wire! Know your loved one and keep a distance between what you feel and what he/she feels. 'Stand together but not too close together' … and 'Let there be spaces in your together-ness … ' Gibran.

   Make space for one another's will to function.

2. Watch out for the 'Does he take sugar syndrome'! Preserve the personhood of the dependent one and avoid controlling the other. Our own self control is what we have been gifted with, and need to work on.

3. My guiding light while caring for David was to look for what he wanted and then go for it. I saw his life like a little boat that was at times stranded on the sandbanks when the tide went out and which needed a chock to keep him steady. Remaining open to what he wanted was very important. He was the best judge of what felt best for him. Towards the end he was in the Hospice once more, weeks before his death; his attitude to being there changed and he clearly wanted to come home. So home he came.

4. The power of gratitude. David was a most undemanding patient. In other words he did not order me about. Obviously his needs were very great latterly and I battled often with exhaustion. But always his gratitude and deep acceptance blew me away and gave me energy to carry on. There is healing power in genuine gratitude rather than just 'being polite', which is civilised but not necessarily heartfelt. As a carer, I made a habit of practising gratitude by looking for God in people, creation, music, art, cooking and food, and there is no end to God's gifts. This helped me to be positive and therefore free (I think) from self-pity which is an enemy to whom to say no.

5. As time went on, I became increasingly aware of the distinction between the body and the spirit. They, with the mind, were clearly joined, yet separate. The spirit needed feeding as much as the body, but feeding with colour and sound and texture. Music was important to us both. We went to concerts when we

could and played CDs at home in the bedroom. As David's body deteriorated and ceased to function normally, without the help of tubes, bags, pills and syringe driver etc, so his spirit shone through the distressing clobber with a strength that ener-gised me and filled me with wonder. He didn't make holy utterances, but just went on loving the best he could. When he died, his body had had it, but his spirit I know was as alive as it ever was. I believe his spirit returned to be united with his Maker. That knowledge comforts me even now, despite the mystery of wondering what is meant by the resurrection of the body when David's body is clearly in ashes in a box under the Cathedral floor!

6. The timing of the prognosis question is important. We both needed to agree about being ready to ask for the prognosis. Losing David was my greatest dread for some years and we put off the prognosis question (David was not a questioner by nature, unlike me) until July 2004, a few months before his death in March 2005. By July 2004, his body was showing increasing signs of deterioration and needing more surgery and medication. So David, Jenny and I met together with the sur-geon and put the question. She told us what she thought. She was spot on. 'You'll probably be here for Christmas, and then, if you're lucky, you'll make it to the Spring.'

After this, the landscape changed for each of us, and we started to prepare in reality for the end-time; for David's death. At the same time we each knew that any of us could go before him. We all have to be ready today. Our lives are in the Lord's hands. Knowledge of the facts enabled us to plan and talk more openly together about the last lap. Living in the Present Moment became very important. This meant living life as nor-mally as possible. It meant accepting the ups and downs as they occurred without complaining, but with an attitude of 'There we go again!' and 'What a palaver!'. It also was important to have our wills up to date and enduring powers of attorney in place. It opened up the way to talk about a funeral too.

7. Facing the reality that the end was near. The battle for life changed to a recognition of the importance of dying well. After the answer to the prognosis question we had hugs and a good weep, releasing a lot of pent-up tension. This was part of the

'letting go' process. On the day we received the prognosis, we decided to have a break, and then meet up and talk later that evening and face the 'What do we feel?' question. David's first response was addressed to me. 'What will you do?' It mattered how I would manage without him. His first thoughts were for me which was very touching. I obviously did not know how it would be, but I still have the list of what I would miss, and of the people that I would be in touch with, and the things that I would enjoy doing after his death and it was a long one! He was glad to know that. Jenny was clearly deeply sad for her boys and for herself, and for me, but she was very positive and sensible. She has always been allergic to sentimentality, which is different of course from pure sentiment. She told David that we would look after each other. That has proved to be true. When I have needed Jenny she has been there. But she is glad that I have a life of my own with friends and neighbours for the day to day contact. We talk on the phone most days and it is wonderful to touch base like that. She dropped everything when my breast cancer diagnosis came through and she was a rock. Just knowing that she was there was a great strength to me. She left me in the hands of my neighbours who were also wonderful. We are there still for each other.

8. Keeping up hobbies and interests. Where possible, this helps to bring some needed balance and gives the mind a rest from worrying. For four years, my primary responsibility was caring for David and concern for his quality of life and his dignity. This also included the responsibility to keep myself fit (I went to the gym at 8 am for 40 mins before breakfast) and living as balanced a life as we could, taking rest when we could, however short, eating a balanced diet and keeping in touch with friends. We both kept up our singing all through his illness. David was keen that I should continue this when he could not, and I was grateful for his encouragement. Singing was like a breath of fresh air and also enabled my patient to know that, even in his need, he was setting me free to meet my needs. He liked to see me enjoying myself and this fed us both. David kept up his love of gardening and he went on painting for as long as possible. Towards the end, he would do a ten-minute weed to get the fresh air, the exercise and the enjoyment. Even now I realise

how that daily ten minutes built up and I miss my weeder! It is important for the patient to feel he/she is contributing something however small. It all adds up, and helps with maintaining dignity and reducing frustration.

9. Keeping a diary. One of the most helpful things for me has been my commitment to my diary or journal. I have kept it since 1985. I write quite fully each night and sometimes at other times. It has become a non-judging friend and a place where I can set down the reality of the day's doings, as well as my feelings. It has also become a vehicle for wonder in which I can get a bit carried away over a thing of beauty. Sometimes it turns into a kind of prayer.

10. Writing letters to each other can be helpful – even when we live together. Thoughts crystallise, and letters can be something to savour. I have come across pages from a long letter I wrote to David, just thanking him for who he was and for the way he adapted to share my life so much more fully in retirement. He set me free in retirement, and shared the domestic routine so wonderfully. I was amazed at the difference it made to me. Equally, I had to be able to let go of my kitchen and the cooking etc. more often! David wanted to free me to write, but he had his own book to publish first. This was a huge commitment and I was virtually his editor. Once his book had been launched, he made a plan to put aside certain days to take on domestic tasks in order to set me free to write. But that was interrupted, as we know.

11. Keeping in touch with friends and family throughout David's illness was hugely important. We did not want to be isolated because we could have drowned in self-pity if we had been denied the love and interest and prayers of family and friends. Keeping in touch involved a good deal of effort and time, keeping David always in the loop. Making a friend of the answer-phone became crucial in keeping the house peaceful and friends informed. It was a necessary discipline for me to switch on the answer phone, instead of trying to answer every phone call as it happened. The answer phone prevented me becoming an Exhausted Butterfly or a Long-Playing Record – saying the same thing over and over and getting nothing else done. Preparing fresh, positive, and factual bulletins to put on

the answer phone each day – sometimes twice a day – enabled me to focus on the positive and to make space for David and me to be quiet together, to entertain visitors without jumping up and down every time the phone rang. It also gave us much to look forward to after yet another chemo trip to the hospital – coming home to listen to our friends' voices and feel their companionship. This use of the answer phone obviously did not stop either of us from ringing back whenever we wanted to. It also protected us from possible unsolicited Press calls. But people are different and some prefer to keep themselves to themselves very much more. I have never regretted 'opening up' despite the effort involved in keeping in touch. Listening to answer phone messages and responding to them forced me to keep reaching out when it might have been tempting to shut the door to the reaching out of others. This would have prevented us from receiving great strength from the love and care that was being held out to us. Some might regard this approach to the phone as self-indulgent. But if Jesus could send the multitudes away when he needed some space, then I reckoned it was ok for us to do the same thing!

12. There is a difference between positive acceptance and negative resignation. David was a very accepting person until it came to big issues of justice etc! He accepted his suffering without being resigned to it. He offered it. This was beautiful to witness. Somehow he knew when it was time to come home from the hospice – to die. There was no panic or upset in the rhythm of living. He lived fully while he could. He was still reading a book during the weeks before his death even though he was drugged and finding it increasingly hard to concentrate. He loved his cricket and enjoyed that on the TV. Cricket became one of the best pain relievers I know. Diversion is an important tool. Too much thinking about 'what next?' and 'what if?' can cause us to drown in our own thoughts, just as too much talking with too many friends can cause confusion. Some like to give advice although it is rarely asked for. It is important to know when to stop.

13. A Safe Place: David and I had separate spiritual directors. They have been people we could trust and respect. Richard was just right for me for all those years before he moved to

Brighton. The time in between – looking for another Richard – was quite stressful. Of course there will never be another Richard. Now I go to a Catholic priest locally whom David and I both knew a little and whom we respected. He has been a lifeline for me. I asked him to help me let David go. He did just that and more. We have always kept our sessions to a strict hour every month on his territory. Each month I write my review for him which is an honest account of how I have been, warts and all. I read it to him, while he puts his feet up and listens before commenting on what he has heard. This way of communicating has helped me to keep my feet on the ground and to be honest, and it enables me to keep up my writing. My spiritual director has been hugely encouraging about that. He has not done my growing up for me. Rather, he has bolstered my will to live and to solve my own problems. He has provided the Christlike companionship that I sought. With him I have felt free to weep and to share my exhaustion during the toughest times. Having a person like that in a place like that means you don't have to spill everything out to everyone all the time, becoming neurotic and confused in the process. Neither do you take it out of your patient in a moment of 'losing it'. This process has helped to clear my head and I know that my spiritual director would tell me if he thought I was not on track. It is wonderful to be told by such a person, in the middle of some crisis ridden days, and even sometimes after tears, 'You're at peace'. It is a safe place and a place where Christ is.

14. Laughter they say is the best medicine. I was reading my diary for 2002 when you both came to stay. It was a happy week, and I have recorded that David told me that Ted always brought the best out of me, which meant I laughed a lot when we were together. And so we did. David had a sense of humour, but he was not a habitual joker. Often we need others around to get us laughing. I occasionally draw cartoons for friends – one being for my 94 year old uncle who told me he found it difficult to adapt to a shower after loving his bath which had been replaced with a shower. He laughed when I suggested singing 'There shall be show-ers of ble-ss-ing' next time he showered. I drew a thick line drawing of him, seated in the shower (suit-

ably screened!) clutching a sponge and singing … He was thrilled and rang up straightaway to say how he loved it and it made him laugh. It helped me to see the funny side of aging too which I hope continues when I can't get in and out of the bath myself.

15. Time with the solicitor: I found this one of the most stressful things of all. David was much better about it. After all he wanted to be a lawyer years ago. Having to get my head around the realities of wills, enduring powers of attorney etc. was very difficult for me. I am so glad I did it with David when he was well. He was such a support here, as he did not panic. Seeing that things are in order while compos mentis and reasonably healthy is important. Otherwise we leave a mess for our children. It is important for peace of mind to have our affairs in order and to share the responsibility early on.

16. Planning a funeral: I didn't feel that David was all that keen to make decisions about this, and on the whole preferred to leave it to me. He and I did not talk very much about our funerals. But his sister, and Jenny, and our rector did talk about the funeral, and plan it together, both before and after David's death. When my mother was declining, we talked in the family about her funeral, expecting it to come many months before it did. At that late stage, she was in no state to engage with funeral plans. It is helpful to one's family to put some things down on paper; ideas of who might take the service and/or contribute or preach; some favourite music or hymns. My father left an ideal two sheets of A4 with details of whom to contact, phone numbers, suggestions about funeral directors. He included bank account numbers, and various little ideas – but without any suggestion that he was controlling us. Because of this, David and I put some thought into preparing something similar for Jenny.

17. Talking about death with the family in short bursts and naturally, releases a lot of pent-up emotion. But it needs to be managed, as it will be more upsetting for some than for others. Some are not ready and should be given an exit route from the conversation. Better to have two sessions that work than one that doesn't. Don't exclude the children.

18. We talked together about the end times, but not in dramatic ways or for too long at any one time. Soon after David's initial diagnosis, we went to London for Colin Cowdrey's Thanksgiving Service in Westminster Abbey. David had been asked to take part in the prayers. He had been offered surgery within a fortnight of the diagnosis but refused because he wanted to keep faith with his commitment to take part in his friend's service. So we lived with this secret for a week or two more, telling only close family and friends. On the way to London in the train, I suggested that we might raise the question of 'What if you died?' on the way back, and discuss it together, in order to begin to open up the issue that lay beneath the surface. David agreed to think about this. On the way back we talked, as planned, for part of the way, and the spell was broken. We knew we could talk about it again at any time without falling apart. To some extent, we had already faced the question of 'What if …?' many years ago when my own cancer was diagnosed. Sometimes David would refer to that time and to my recovery, saying how much this previous encounter with cancer had helped him to be aware that there was still life to be lived despite the diagnosis.

19. In the end, God. Towards the end of his life David continued to have private sessions with his spiritual director (Brian). Then we would have a meal all together. During his last visit, Brian left a quote with us: 'He who can say, "In the end, God", has a strength that is unfathomable.' We both believed David was returning to God – the final Homecoming. He was not, apparently, longing to get there, because he knew he was loved down here and he wanted to live. But his relationship with God was such that he did not appear to be afraid to let go to God at the end. He was at peace. The morphine was helping too. My *final* challenge was to let him go in words, as well as in my heart and in my head. I had to tell him that I was ready to let him go to the one who loved us both more than we loved each other. This was incredibly hard for me, but I said it and I meant it. David died in minutes after that. Just before that moment, Jenny's final words had been: 'We'll look after each other, Dad'. This was music to David's ears, I am sure, as it was to mine. The nurse told us we could not have said two more

helpful things to help him to let go of us. As you know, this was soon after the end of my birthday party which he had wanted to be there for.

20. Much of my survival as a carer and then as a bereaved person has been due to making decisions quite quickly. I have been increasingly conscious that there is so often a fork in the road. I must choose which road to take – the negative or the positive – without dithering. If I start to wobble between two options, this upsets the business of living. What do you want to do? and, 'Which road do you want to take?' are questions that demand action. These questions had to be answered and then I would find peace and stability. Decisions are a way of turning uncertainty into certainty. There's nothing actually wrong with dithering. It is just very uncomfortable and can be dealt with by deciding what we actually want to do. After David's death I wanted to be positive as I had so much to be thankful for. Too much thinking and analysing can upset the 'doing'. Too little thinking and analysing leads to knee jerk decisions at an highly emotional time.

21. Praying together. David and I always prayed together every night before sleep. We almost always managed to sort out any arguments before the sun went down. David said Morning Prayer every morning too. We used to say this together. But after some thought I stopped doing this with him. Part of me regrets this, and part of me knows that it was right at the time. I already had my own quiet time which took a different form – slightly more non-conformist. Latterly, when David was very weary and ill he was happy for me to read something short to him from my little book of meditations by Ruth Etchells (*Just as I Am*) at night, before we prayed. This little book has sustained me for nearly 15 years. We would always stop and say a brief prayer before setting off for another chemo or hospital appointment. Something like, 'Here we go Lord, off on another adventure. Please stay with us and help us look for you in everyone we meet.' In this way, the relationship with the Lord became more like breathing than ever. Similarly before meals, we would say 'thank you' in our own way. At night we would sometimes sing, 'Glory to Thee my God this night,' or 'Lord keep us safe this night,' or say Compline together.

22. Keep up with church friends. They care and will pray and offer help.

23. Make a list of those who offer help and phone numbers and use it shamelessly. People really do want to help. Don't ask people you do not feel at ease with, or mistrust. I still have my list eight years later!

    e.g. Jim – shopping … tel no
    Brenda – driving … tel no
    Val – anything, day or night … tel no etc.

24. Learning to live with uncertainty. This was difficult at times. Even the consultants said sometimes that they did not always know what was going wrong. We felt this was rather touching and humble, instead of them making something up to keep the patient relatively content by giving a label. We never knew how David would die, or when, until the very end. We had to learn to live with that and to accept it: to be patient. So it was time to concentrate on what we did know. Bill Vanstone talks about Christ's active passivity in *The Stature of Waiting*. Working on patience was very important as there was a lot of waiting around; a lot of unknowing. Concentrating on the quality of life became important: seeing the people David wanted to see; visiting places he wanted to visit; new pyjamas from time to time; taking trouble over food preparation, little treats and keeping the home a place of peace and fun. All these seemed to count for something. A short walk to the beach together and sitting on a bench saying nothing, but holding hands – all these little things helped towards the final good-bye. Children were a boon bringing a natural lightness with them. The grandchildren were always a joy.

25. Agree or not beforehand to see a consultant together. Don't be taken by surprise. Take a notebook with the questions you want to ask, but take care to let the patient call the tune.

26. Get to know your local hospice. Pay a visit well before you need it. You may never need it! See what they offer. Jenny and I were fairly ignorant. Visiting the hospice before it was needed, opened our eyes and reassured us for when it became a reality. 'It's perfect', said Jenny. We could then share our confidence and knowledge with David.

27. Look after yourself. Keep taking trouble with your appear-ance. Don't let yourself go. Eat proper meals unhurriedly when possible. Take rests in short bursts as you will get very tired. I set the alarm clock sometimes for 10 minutes for instance, then you can really let go.

28. Intimacy. This is so important to maintain long after the libido has gone. Holding hands unhurriedly, and sitting, and lying together and being close in so many gentle physical ways became precious. But even some of these can be overdone and there needed to be good communicating, and knowing when to stop. Even helping him on and off the commode in the early hours of the morning became almost a little dance – a little do-si-do. The warm flannel when washing his face I know he loved. Brushing hair (until it all came out) and cutting toenails … these things can carry love as much as anything.

That is quite enough! I am sure I have left out so much. You will know most of this already. This is an unedited flow yet I hope some of it will help with your own journey together. I have laid it out so that you can scribble notes on the right hand side if you want to.

Let me know how you get on.

With my love, Grace

Notes

1   T. S. Eliot, 'East Coker', *Four Quartets*, London: Faber and Faber, 1944, p. 23.
2   Archbishop John Sentamu, at his inauguration as Archbishop of York.
3   The Rt Revd Hugh Gough.
4   Gerard W. Hughes, *God of Surprises*, London: Darton, Longman and Todd, 1985.
5   Peter McGovern, and recorded by The Spinners.
6   Amy Carmichael, *His Thoughts Said ... His Father Said ...*, London: SPCK, 1941.
7   Catholic Agency for Overseas Development.
8   Grace Sheppard, *An Aspect of Fear*, London: Darton, Longman and Todd, 1989.
9   Khalil Gibran, 'Marriage' in *The Prophet*, London: William Heinemann Ltd, 1926.
10 Canon Brian McConnell.
11 John Baillie, *A Diary of Private Prayer*, Oxford: Oxford University Press, 1936.
12 George Eliot, *The Mill on the Floss*, Penguin Classics.
13 Ruth Etchells, *Just As I Am: Personal Prayers for Every Day*, London: SPCK, 1994.
14 Richard Gillard, *The Servant Song*, © 1977 Scripture in Song/ Maranatha!Music. Administered by Song Solutions CopyCare, 14 Horsted Square, Uckfield, TN22 1QG. info@songsolutions.org. Used by permission.
15 See Appendix 1.
16 David Sheppard, *Steps Along Hope Street: My Life in London and Liverpool*, London: Hodder and Stoughton, 2002.
17 Professor Higgins, from the musical *My Fair Lady*.
18 Jo's Trust was set up after her death for those involved with cervical cancer. This can be accessed online at www.jostrust.co.uk
19 Psalm 139.8–10, RSV.
20 Deuteronomy 33.27.
21 John V. Taylor, *A Matter of Life and Death*, London: SCM Press, 1986.

22 James Houston, *The Transforming Power of Prayer: Deepening your Friendship with God*, Oxford: Lion, 1989.

23 Thanksgiving prayer in Church of England Communion Service.

24 Canon Brian McConnell.

25 Henri Nouwen, *Here and Now: Living in the Spirit*, London: Darton, Longman and Todd, 1994.

26 Rabindranath Tagore.

27 Source unknown.

28 Brian Wren, reproduced from 'Piece Together Praise' by permission of Stainer & Bell Ltd, London, England. www.stainer.co.uk

29 Later Dean of Chichester.

30 Kahlil Gibran, 'Friendship' in *The Prophet*, London: William Heinemann Ltd, 1926.

31 Source unknown.

32 James Houston, *The Transforming Power of Prayer: Deepening your Friendship with God*, Oxford: Lion, 1989.

33 Frank Topping, *Lord of Life*, London: Lutterworth Press, 1982.

34 Archbishop Desmond Tutu.

35 T. S. Eliot, 'East Coker', *Four Quartets*, London: Faber and Faber, 1944, p. 22.

36 Eric James, *In the House of My Friends*, London: Continuum, 2003.

Bibliography

Peter Atkinson, *Friendship and the Body of Christ*, London: SPCK, 2004.

Warren R. Bardsley, *Touched by Grace: Walking the Path of Grief*, Church in the Marketplace, 2005.

Shirley du Boulay, *Cicely Saunders: The Founder of the Modern Hospice Movement*, London: Hodder and Stoughton, 1984.

Amy Carmichael, *His Thoughts Said ... His Father Said ...*, London: SPCK, 1941.

John Cornwell, *Darwin's Angel: An Angelic Riposte to* The God Delusion, London: Profile Books, 2008.

Jack Dominian, *One like Us: A Psychological Interpretation of Jesus*, London: Darton, Longman and Todd, 1998.

Ruth Etchells, *Just As I Am: Personal Prayers for Every Day*, London: SPCK, 1994.

Eric Fromm, *The Art of Loving*, London: Mandala/Unwin, 1957.

Kahlil Gibran, *The Prophet*, London: Heinemann Publishing Ltd, 1926.

Dag Hammarskjöld, *Markings*, London: Faber and Faber, 1964.

James Houston, *The Transforming Power of Prayer: Deepening your Friendship with God*, Oxford: Lion, 1989.

Gerard W. Hughes, *God of Surprises*, London: Darton, Longman and Todd, 1985.

Christopher Jamison, *Finding Sanctuary: Monastic Steps for Everyday Life*, London: Weidenfeld and Nicolson, 2006.

Eric James, *In the House of My Friends*, London: Continuum, 2003.

James Jones, *Jesus and the Earth*, London: SPCK, 2003.

Michael Mayne, *The Enduring Melody*, London: Darton, Longman and Todd, 2006.

Jürgen Moltmann, *The Church in the Power of the Spirit*, London: SCM Press, 1977.

Henri Nouwen, *In the House of the Lord*, London: Darton, Longman and Todd, 1986.

Henri Nouwen, *Here and Now*, London: Darton, Longman and Todd, 1994.

M. Scott Peck, *The Road Less Travelled*, London: Rider, 1978.

Ray Pahl, *On Friendship*, Cambridge: Polity Press, 2000.

Joyce Rupp, *May I have This Dance?*, Notre Dame IN: Ave Maria Press, 1992.

Charles Smyth, *The Friendship of Christ*, Cambridge: Longmans, Green & Co Ltd, 1945.

Brian Thorne, *Behold the Man: A Therapist's Meditations on the Passion of Jesus Christ*, London: Darton, Longman and Todd, 1991.

John V. Taylor, *A Matter of Life and Death*, London: SCM Press, 1986.

W. H. Vanstone, *The Stature of Waiting*, London: Darton, Longman and Todd, 1982.

W. H. Vanstone, *Fare Well in Christ*, London: Darton, Longman and Todd, 1997.

Michael Wenham, *My Donkey Body*, Oxford: Monarch, 2008.

Harry Williams, *The True Wilderness*, London: Constable, 1965.